ACCLA
WHAT YOUR DOCT
YOU A
ALZHEIMER'S DISEASE

"Highly recommended. . . . Dr. Devi helps take the fear, pain, and suffering out of Alzheimer's."

—Dharma Singh Khalsa, M.D., president/medical director, Alzheimer's Prevention Foundation International, and author of *The Better Memory Kit*

"This book empowers every family to become its own best advocate. Among Dr. Devi's many accomplishments, this may well be her finest. I suspect many doctors are going to (secretly) read it, too!"

—P. Murali Doraiswamy, M.D., senior fellow, Center for the Study of Aging, Duke University Medical Center

"An important contribution. . . . In a clear and surprisingly upbeat fashion, Dr. Devi discusses the symptoms, diagnosis, prevention, and management of Alzheimer's disease. . . . This book should find its way to every household."

—Lila A. Wallis, M.D., M.A.C.P., clinical professor of medicine, Weill Medical College of Cornell University, and founding president, The National Council on Women's Health

"Dr. Devi's groundbreaking research helps to allay the great fear of memory loss. Easy to read and packed with preventive measures, this is the book millions of baby boomers have been waiting for—for ourselves and our parents."

—Susan L. Taylor, editorial director, *Essence*

WHAT YOUR DOCTOR MAY *NOT* TELL YOU ABOUT™ ALZHEIMER'S DISEASE

The Complete Guide to Preventing, Treating, and Coping with Memory Loss

GAYATRI DEVI, M.D.
and Deborah Mitchell

A Lynn Sonberg Book

WARNER BOOKS

NEW YORK BOSTON

This book is derived from the personal clinical and research experience of the author, as well as the author's interpretation of available research in the field. The author is not engaged in rendering professional advice or services to the individual reader, and the suggestions in this book are in no way a substitute for a medical evaluation and recommendations by a physician. All matters concerning your health require ongoing medical supervision. Thus, the author and publisher do not recommend changing your medication or hormone replacement regimen without consulting your physician. The author and publisher are not liable or responsible for any direct loss or damage allegedly arising from any information or suggestion in this book or from the use of any treatments mentioned in the book.

Warner Books

Time Warner Book Group
1271 Avenue of the Americas, New York, NY 10020
Visit our Web site at www.twbookmark.com.

Printed in the United States of America

First Printing: November 2004
10 9 8 7 6 5 4 3 2 1

Library of Congress Cataloging-in-Publication Data
Devi, Gayatri.
What your doctor may not tell you about Alzheimer's disease : the complete guide to preventing, treating, and coping with memory loss / by Gayatri Devi and Deborah Mitchell.
p. cm.
"A Lynn Sonberg Book."
Includes bibliographical references and index.
ISBN 0-446-69188-7
1. Alzheimer's disease—Popular works. 2. Alzheimer's disease—Prevention—Popular works. I. Mitchell, Deborah R. II. Title.
RC523.2.D486 2004
616.8'31—dc22 2004006632

Cover design by Diane Luger
Book design by Charles A. Sutherland

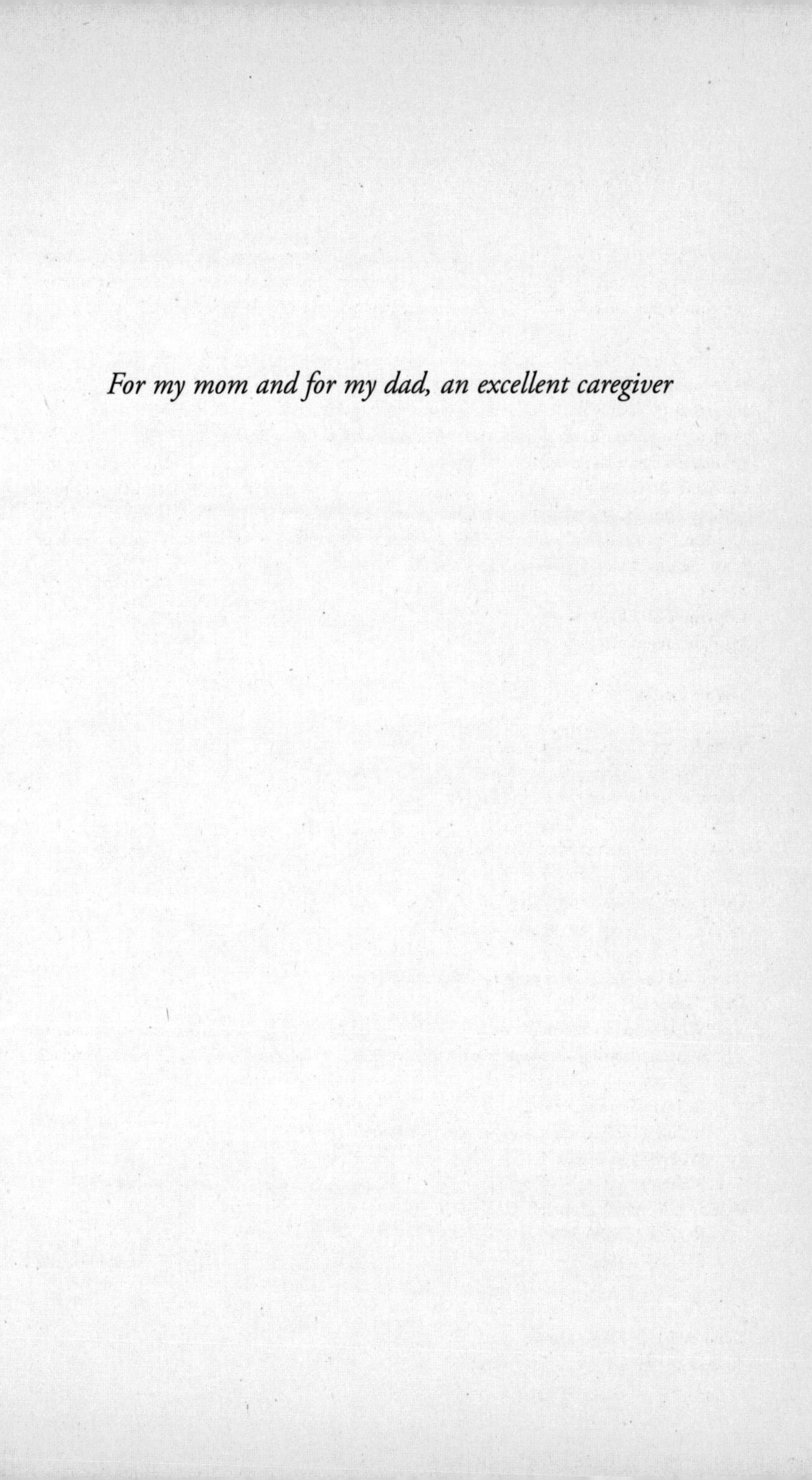

For my mom and for my dad, an excellent caregiver

Contents

What Your Doctor May *Not* Tell You About™ Alzheimer's Disease

Introduction

The sword of Damocles hangs over the heads of the many people who suffer from memory problems: a diagnosis of Alzheimer's disease. The phrase, rarely spoken, is so dreaded that many delay seeking help because they worry their worst fears will be confirmed. Yet even if you or your loved one do hear those words from your doctor, it is critically important that you know there is hope—that early diagnosis and treatment can do so much to treat memory loss and slow its progress, whether due to Alzheimer's disease or to another of the many conditions that mimic the disease. Or if you're worried about getting Alzheimer's disease sometime in the future, you should also know that research points to preventive measures that everyone can take—ones that can easily be incorporated into your daily routine—that can help prevent memory loss and reduce the odds that the disease will ever develop.

We have seen how education, raised awareness, and early detection have changed the landscape of breast cancer. I believe Alzheimer's disease is poised for a similar breakthrough. By practicing early diagnosis and treatment of memory disorders and Alzheimer's disease, the quality of life of the nearly

360,000 Americans who will be diagnosed with the disease this year will be vastly improved.

In the course of a decade, I have worked with thousands of individuals and caregivers affected by Alzheimer's disease. A striking thing I have observed is that patients and their families have many unvoiced anxieties. These pent-up fears can get in the way of patients being able to enjoy the fulfilling, independent life they deserve. These fears can also be greatly reduced once people are shown ways they can take back some control of the disease and their lives. That's why in this book I would like to share with you not only my approach for diagnosis and treatment, but more importantly, the stories of hope, courage, and love that I've had the privilege to experience during my years of working with people who have Alzheimer's disease. I also want to share how you can make modest changes in your lifestyle—practicing mental exercises, taking antioxidants, getting enough sleep, reducing stress, exercising, and considering natural hormone replacement therapy—that can help prevent memory loss and Alzheimer's disease.

One of the biggest misconceptions about this disease is that affected persons and their families can't do anything about it. Time after time, people come to me harboring such feelings of defeat, often ready to give up even before they begin the fight. They've read, they've heard, they've been led to believe that once people get Alzheimer's disease, their lives are over.

Thankfully, they are wrong. And this book shows them what they can do about it, by offering tools that allow people with Alzheimer's disease to be as independent and to live as dignified a life as possible.

Yes, Alzheimer's disease is a progressive condition that can be potentially devastating, but the course of the illness varies from person to person. Every day I see individuals with Alzheimer's who are functioning independently and who have been doing so for significant periods of time. The stereotype of the patient in a nursing home, a shell of their former self, is true in only a minority of patients. The truth is that most patients live at home with dignity and a measure of that treasured value, independence. It is my firm belief—and my experience—that the vast majority of patients can do so with appropriate treatment, education, and support. The symptoms of Alzheimer's can be managed effectively using a combination of medications and behavioral methods and by continuing to stimulate the mind in ways that are enjoyable and effective. I have found this method to help individuals live rewarding lives up until their death. In this book, I will share some of their stories and how these people get the most from each and every day.

The irony is that even with far more aggressive and inevitably fatal conditions like malignant tumors, patients are more proactive about seeking help and undergoing exhaustive treatments, often to prolong life by only a few months. Yet for patients who have Alzheimer's disease, they can harvest *years* of quality time if they take the steps that are outlined in this book.

Here, we share hope and an understanding of Alzheimer's disease with you and others who are searching for guidance and support. We explain how you can help your loved one have more control of his or her life and live with joy and peace instead of fear and despair, and how you can work with your physicians to ensure that quality of life is maintained for as long as possible.

We begin our journey by addressing the burning questions so many people have, such as, "What causes memory problems?", "How do I know if I have Alzheimer's disease?", "What causes Alzheimer's disease?", "How do I find a qualified doctor to help me?", "How can I prevent memory loss and Alzheimer's disease?", and "What role do hormones play in memory loss?" The answers to all these questions are important, but the last is of particular interest to women, especially because most doctors don't address this critical issue.

Although you may be tempted to jump ahead to the second part of the book, where I offer practical, hands-on ways to handle the challenges of Alzheimer's disease and memory loss, I urge you to read the opening chapters that explore these questions. The answers provide not only a wealth of up-to-date information and tips, but also lay the groundwork for the chapters that follow, a foundation that will make your journey and that of the person with Alzheimer's disease an easier one.

The soul of the book, so to speak, is contained in the second part of the book, where I explain treatment approaches, lifestyle changes, and caregiver guidelines that you and your loved one can incorporate into your lives to make them as fulfilling and loving as possible. I know from experience that these methods work, and I will share with you many stories of individuals with Alzheimer's and their loved ones who use them and who continue to flourish in the face of this disease.

"Brain boosters" are what I call some of the most useful and enjoyable approaches I use in my practice. These are mental exercises that can be performed at home (or, in a few cases, while out walking or shopping), using common supplies. These exercises are useful both for people who have Alzheimer's disease and, in many cases, for those who want to preserve their memory and help prevent Alzheimer's disease. This book offers you dozens of brain boosters, with complete instructions, and you can choose the ones to incorporate into your life or the life of your loved one.

While exercising the mind is critically important, it is also essential to nurture the mind-body connection. Given the complexity of Alzheimer's disease, I find that the most effective treatment requires a multifaceted approach, using a combination of multiple drugs, aggressive treatment of common medical problems like heart disease and diabetes, and alternative approaches, such as nutritional supplements, herbal remedies, and natural hormones. I explain how you can work with your doctor and at home to make these approaches a part of your life.

Eric Kandel, a Nobel Prize winner for his work on memory, has stated that a cure for Alzheimer's will be found within the next five years, which places it before the end of this decade (2010), and this level of confidence from a giant in the field is heartening. I share his optimism. In the last decade alone, four new drugs were approved by the Food and Drug Administration for treating Alzheimer's disease, and in the new millennium a fifth was added to the list. Several others are in the pipeline.

I cannot yet offer you a cure, but in this book I can share with you my approach that will allow people with Alzheimer's disease and their loved ones to experience rewarding and meaningful lives. My wish is that the information in this book will help enhance the lives of those who have Alzheimer's disease and encourage the hearts and spirits of those who care for them.

PART I

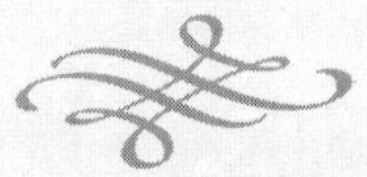

ALZHEIMER'S DISEASE
AND
THE BRAIN

Chapter 1

The Brain, Memory, and Alzheimer's Disease

Perhaps the biggest mystery that faces humankind is not whether there is life on other planets or how the universe began, but exactly how the human brain works. I believe the human brain is the last frontier. What is thought? What is memory? How is memory stored? Where is memory stored? What happens when memory is lost? How does the brain know how to manage this concept we call memory?

You probably had not thought much about these questions until now. But, because you have picked up this book, things have probably changed. Now you want some answers—which we will provide in this chapter—because either you or a loved one is having memory "problems." Keys are being misplaced, again and again. The names of neighbors are being forgotten. Perhaps bills aren't paid on time or are forgotten altogether. The titles of favorite books can't be recalled. And somewhere in the back of your mind, two words loom, even though they frighten you and you try to push them away:

Alzheimer's disease.

And to that we reply, don't be alarmed. Why?

- Some forgetfulness occurs as a natural part of aging. There is a difference between this age-related forgetfulness and the memory loss associated with Alzheimer's disease and other forms of dementia. I will talk about the differences in the pages ahead.
- If you are concerned about memory loss, there are things you can do to help prevent it. (These are discussed in chapter 6.)
- And, if Alzheimer's disease is diagnosed, there are many ways to make the life of the person who has the disease a loving, rich, and fulfilling one.

There is much confusion and apprehension surrounding what constitutes "normal" age-related memory loss and changes in brain function and what clues suggest the serious and progressive memory loss that is characteristic of Alzheimer's disease. To help alleviate any anxiety and fears you may have about memory loss and to help you more clearly understand what Alzheimer's disease is, I believe it is important for you to have a basic understanding of the following:

- healthy brain activity and how the brain ages normally;
- how memory works and what constitutes normal age-related memory loss;
- the signs and symptoms of Alzheimer's disease and other forms of dementia; and
- how the normal age-related changes in brain function and memory compare with those associated with Alzheimer's disease.

Perhaps more than any other medical condition, Alzheimer's disease has a profound impact not only on the individuals who have the disease, but on their family, friends, and other significant people in their lives. I believe it is essential that those who are closest to the people who have Alzheimer's understand that the changes in personality and behavior they will witness and experience are the result of physical damage to the brain, and that this damage leads to much frustration, anxiety, and fear on the part of those who have the disease *and* those who love them.

Individuals who are affected by Alzheimer's are *not* their disease; they are not Alzheimer's patients—they are people affected by Alzheimer's disease. They are still mother, father, sister, brother, aunt, uncle, grandmother, best friend; they are still individuals capable of loving and sharing; they still need a hug and a smile. So do you. And you'll be better able to give and receive those feelings once you become more familiar with your challenger—the human brain and the changes it can go through during this disease process.

NORMAL BRAIN ACTIVITY

The human brain is without question the most complex piece of machinery known to humankind. It contains an estimated 100 billion nerve cells that tirelessly communicate and make it possible for you to think, remember, move, perform vital functions, and, overall, experience life. Your brain controls virtually every aspect of your life, from sitting and breathing to your desire to eat or paint, to your empathy for a friend or your joy in seeing a sunset.

Looking Inside a Healthy Brain

Even though the brain is such a complex organ, we are understanding it more and more through research, which is also helping us uncover the mysteries of why memory loss, Alzheimer's disease, and other dementias occur. I believe a basic understanding of how a healthy brain functions can help you better appreciate what happens to people who experience memory loss or dementia. It will also help you understand how the "brain boosters" (discussed in chapter 6) can benefit you and your loved ones.

The human brain, although weighing in at a mere three and a half pounds, is very much a heavyweight. Nearly half of all the blood pumped from the heart goes directly to the brain, even though this organ accounts for a mere fraction of the entire body weight. A constant supply of sugar (glucose) is produced by the body at all times to keep the brain nourished. Why does the brain need all this energy? The billions of nerve cells are in constant activity, whether you are awake or asleep, constantly producing electrical signals. Thanks to new imaging techniques, activity in areas of the brain as small as a grapeseed or as large as an orange can be measured as various tasks are performed.

Different parts of the brain specialize in different tasks, recruiting other areas as needed to best accomplish a given job. While extremely efficient, this level of subspecialization comes at a price. Destruction of an area important for, say, memory or for math will make it difficult for a person to be able to designate another area of their brain to do the same function. Children have this capacity, as their brains are not yet fully developed, but adults are more restricted. Despite this, adults are capable of a tremendous amount of adaptation or "plasticity," so there is some measure of this in our older years as well.

The brain is divided into two sides, or hemispheres. The left side deals with language and details and is the more "analytical" or "logical" part of the brain. The right side deals with space and understanding emotions and is the more "artistic" part of the brain. So, the right side sees the forest, while the left side sees the trees. Some people are more "left brained" while others are more "right brained," yet others are about equal.

If you are wondering which side of your brain you tend to use more, try this experiment. Look quickly (for about one second) at the picture below, then look away.

iiiiiiiiiiiiiiiiiiiiiiiiiiiiiiiiiiiiiiiiiii
iiiii
iiiii
iiiiiiiiiiiiiiiiiiiii
iiiii
iiiii
iiiiiiiiiiiiiiiiiiiiiiiiiiiiiiiiiiiiiiiiiii

What did you see? If you saw the E, you are a right-brainer; if you saw a bunch of little i's, then you are a left-brainer; and if you saw both, you are using both sides of your brain.

Within each side of the brain are various lobes. The frontal lobe, the largest area of the brain, is concerned with voluntary movement, language expression, social judgment, personality, problem solving, and abstract thinking in general. The temporal lobe is involved with memory, language comprehension, and perception. Deep within the temporal lobe is a structure called the hippocampus that can be viewed as a gateway for storing and retrieving certain types of memory. The parietal lobe is important for sensation and for understanding spatial relations. The occipital lobe is involved in vision. (See Figure 1.)

In Alzheimer's disease, the earliest changes occur in the hippocampus and then spread to other areas of the brain,

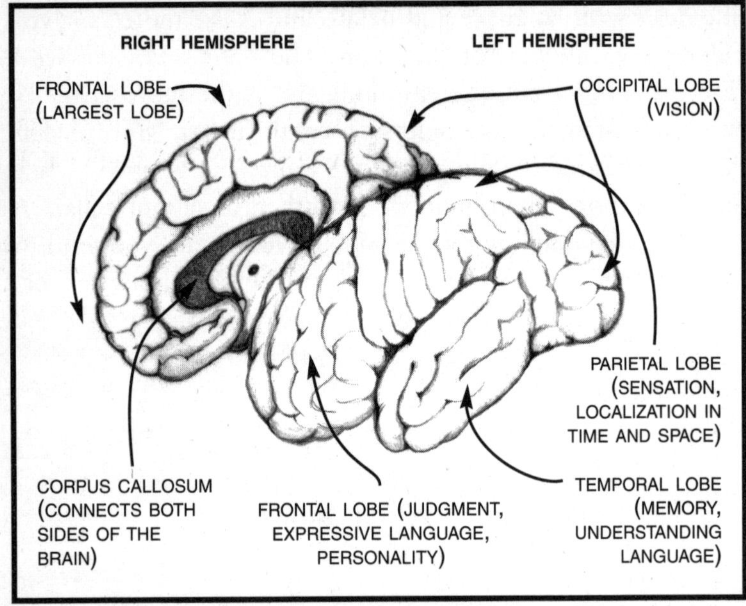

Figure 1: Brain pulled apart in halves

especially the temporal and parietal lobes. The hippocampus is a tiny, sea horse–shaped organ that is one of the most sensitive parts of the brain. It is more vulnerable to the effects of reduced oxygen and glucose supply than any other part. It lies near the middle of the brain, one hippocampus on the right side and another on the left. This organ is very important for the "when," "what," and "where" memories.

It would be helpful if all the brain's functions and tasks were as neatly compartmentalized into the various regions and lobes I've just identified. In reality, however, that isn't so. Memory, for example, isn't confined to just one area of the brain. When we recover a memory, it is as if we cast a net over the entire brain and pull out aspects of the memory from different parts of the brain to form the whole mosaic of the memory. When you hear a snippet of a song, it activates a part of a memory trace, and the brain then may recall for you who you danced with the first time you heard the song, what you were wearing, what your partner's perfume smelled like, and how their skin felt. Each of these bits of the memory mosaic comes from a different part of the brain.

Storage of memory also occurs in the same fashion. For example, when you see and smell a flower, the messages regarding what you see are active in one part of your brain, while the smell is processed in another, and the sorting and filing of the memory of the flower happen in yet another region.

Brain Talk: How Brain Cells Communicate

Neurons and neurotransmitters are the great communicators in the brain. The 100 billion nerve cells in the brain communicate by producing and sending electrical signals to other cells. Unlike heart cells, no two nerve cells actually communicate by direct contact. Instead, when one neuron is ready to communicate with another neuron, a signal travels along the body and axon (a single branch that extends from the neuron's main body; its job is to carry signals to other neurons) (see Figure 2). When a message reaches the tip of the axon, it triggers the release of chemicals called neurotransmitters into the synapse, the space between the axon of the sending neuron and a receiving neuron. The neurotransmitters then attach themselves to receptors (docking sites) on the dendrites (receiving arms) of the receiving neuron. Once the neurotransmitters are attached, the process of sending the signals begins again.

In a healthy brain, a message is transmitted from neuron to neuron until it reaches its intended destination, which may be leg muscles, lungs, eyes, or another part of the brain. Nerve cells are sending signals every second of your life: when you see

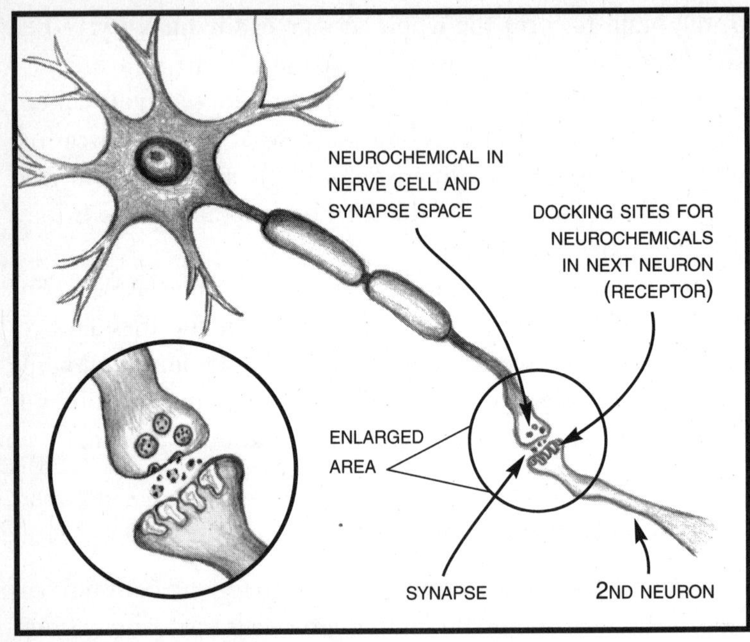

Figure 2: Neuron with a synapse

a flower, stub your toe, fall in love, or digest your lunch, signals are flying.

One way to imagine the brain is to think of it as a very intricate orchestra consisting of billions of positions, all under one conductor (you!), but divided into different sections—strings, reeds, and so on. When one area does not function well or is not in sync with the others, then the music is not quite right, *the mind isn't quite right,* and memory can be affected.

In a healthy brain, nerve cells and neurotransmitters go about their communication function with few or no problems. However, as you'll learn in the next chapter, something interferes with the normal functioning of the neurons and neurotransmitters in people who have Alzheimer's disease.

THE HEALTHY AGING BRAIN AND DECLINING MEMORY

As we age, we expect to feel a few aches and pains and notice graying hair and wrinkles, but these are just the external signs of aging. What about internal changes, particularly in the brain?

The passing of the years is accompanied by a normal dying off of nerve cells in the brain. In fact, brain cells begin to die when people are in their twenties, decades before they even *think* about the possibility of Alzheimer's disease. At the same time, aging is also associated with a decline in the number of synapses (fewer cells means fewer synapses), a decline in the amount of some brain chemicals, and shrinkage of the brain size, often called atrophy. Although we place such a premium on remembering, it is important to realize that *the human brain was designed to forget.* We have evolved over millennia with forgetfulness programmed into our brain as a normal function so that there will be available space for new memories as old memories are pruned away. In some very rare instances, individuals are unable to forget anything. In these situations the person becomes unable to function as the brain becomes clogged with millions of memory traces.

"Senior Moments"

For the majority of people sixty-five years and older, all of these brain changes work together to result in mild forgetfulness, a slight loss of concentration, and a slower response time when, say, they try to recall a telephone number or someone's birthday. They may occasionally forget what to buy at the grocery store, where they put their keys, or the name of the teller they always see at the bank. And, for this majority, these transient episodes of forgetfulness can be annoying, yet certainly manageable.

Sylvia, a sixty-nine-year-old retired accountant, calls her minor slips of memory "senior moments." She finds that making simple adjustments, such as always making a shopping list instead of relying on remembering what she needs from the store, or always putting her car keys in a basket by the front door, has reduced her number of senior moments, as well as stressful episodes. She also keeps her mind active (see chapter 6 for suggestions) by reading and staying socially active as a volunteer in the community.

Memory Loss Is Inevitable but Alzheimer's Is Not

It's important to remember that while all of us will forget more as we get older, loss of memory is not synonymous with Alzheimer's disease or dementia. Many people in their eighties and nineties remain mentally sharp and witty and continue to contribute to society as writers, grandparents, researchers, volunteers, physicians, politicians, and artists. Exactly why some people retain their memories while others do not is still a mystery, but one that researchers and physicians are exploring vigorously.

In fact, contrary to what experts thought for years, recent research is showing us that people can maintain brain plasticity and number of synapses well into their eighties and nineties. This ability doesn't come without some effort, however. Thus the adage "use it or lose it" applies here, and we'll help you do just that in chapter 6, "Brain Boosters: An Exercise Program for Mental Fitness."

WHAT IS MEMORY?

How Are Memories Stored?

Each time you remember something, up to three steps may occur. The first step is your perception or registration of the object or event. Let's say you decide to learn French and you have a list of ten vocabulary words. You look at the words and say them out loud, which allows your senses to register the sight and sound of the words. This is a rapid assessment process, which takes less than a second for each sound. You have created a sensory memory.

In step two, you retain the sensory memory. This typically involves thinking about the words, repeating them several times in class or at home. At this point, this sensory memory is "stored" in short-term memory. However, if you drop out of the French class or don't practice the words over and over again, your memory of them will eventually be replaced by other, incoming memories. The vast majority of short-term memories doesn't make it to the third step (see below), because they aren't important enough to remember for a longer length of time or they were not *consolidated* (practiced, reviewed repeatedly in the mind, or in some other way often brought to your attention). **Short-term memory** is an important concept for people who have Alzheimer's disease, as this is one type of memory that is lost.

In step three, you recall the situation. Not all memories reach this stage. If you stay in your French class, do your homework, and practice speaking French, you will likely remember the words and continue to improve your vocabulary. This memory has been stored in **long-term memory**. Truly long-term memory is always associated with permanent structural changes in nerve cells and circuitry. It is remarkably resistant to destruction. This is why even people who have advanced Alzheimer's disease, who do not know where they are or the names of family members, will give you their parents' names and sing along to old familiar tunes.

All long-term memory is always associated with physical changes in the brain. Physical changes result when nerve cells sprout to form more branches for more connections to other cells, and from the strengthening or weakening of connections between some nerve cells. This type of preferential connecting allows the formation of a pathway or a network. This allows cells with similar functions to establish strong connections with one another, in, for instance, a visual pathway for sight memories and an auditory pathway for sound memories.

On the Types of Memory

I can't think and hit at the same time.
—Yogi Berra

We can also view memory as procedural or declarative. **Declarative memory** is the type of memory that most people associate with having a good memory, that is, the ability to recite facts. Declarative memory is the memory of facts and events; people with a good declarative memory are often good at games such as Trivial Pursuit or *Jeopardy.* This is the kind of memory that is involved in answering "what," "where," and "when" questions. **Procedural memory** is the memory necessary to perform activities like walking, driving, and dancing. It is the answer to a "how" question, as in "How do you walk?" The "when" and "where" answers, which relate to a specific time and place, are far more sensitive to destruction. These memories are affected first in memory disorders.

Constant repetition of an initially declarative memory task such as the multiplication tables or playing the piano makes it a procedural or muscle memory. Think of a skill such as learning to drive. At first, it is a very conscious and describable process, but with repetition it soon becomes automatic and "reflexive." In the process, the brain converts a fragile memory into something very resistant to destruction. Hence, the old adage of habits first being cobwebs, then cables, is true in neuroscience. The brain lays down strong connections between appropriate regions when a task is repeated over and over again.

Great athletes often have very well-developed procedural memories for golf or shooting baskets, for example. Because a lot of their memory is procedural, it is hard for them to describe their skill and teach it to someone else. They play by "instinct." This is why it is sometimes hard for champion athletes to become good coaches. The inimitable Yogi Berra noted the difference between these two forms of memory: "I can't think [declarative memory] and hit [procedural 'muscle' memory] at the same time." By the way, it should come as no surprise that Yogi did not make it as a coach!

Among people who develop Alzheimer's disease, they will first experience destruction of their declarative memory skills, such as what happened when and where (what movie did I see and who was in it), and then the retention of facts (what is the capital of Italy and what is 6 times 6). Very old memories, which occurred when a patient was young, are resistant to destruction. The "when" and "where" memories are destroyed first, the "what" next, and finally the "how" memory is destroyed. Thus persons with abnormal forgetfulness will progress from "When did I last have a sandwich?" and "Where did I put my sandwich?" to "What is a sandwich?" to "How do I eat a sandwich?"

Procedural skills are the most resilient, so that the ability to do whatever it is the person is skilled at, be it cooking or knitting or drafting, is the last to go. In a certain condition called apraxia (an inability to perform purposeful movements), some kinds of manual tasks are affected. In addition to memory changes, in a condition called aphasia, patients will have difficulty with language, although their memory may be intact.

Emotion and Memory

Intense emotions are often associated with unforgettable memories. Thus, neither war experiences nor first kisses are usually forgotten. For such occasions, people often remember the dress they were wearing on the day, what the day was like, about what time of the day it was, what the weather was like, and the surroundings—almost like a snapshot. This is because the part of the brain that controls emotion, a small brain organ called the amygdala, is very closely linked to the hippocampus, which is so important for memory. Various studies have found that memories that have emotional meaning are better laid down in the brain and better retrieved than those that lack emotional significance.

Flashbacks are negative consequences of this emotionally etched memory, where victims of extreme trauma, like war, relive the entire experience in excruciating detail. Seemingly innocuous triggers can set off this emotionally highly sensitive and well-remembered memory trace: a scent in the environment, the color of someone's eyes, the shape of a room, or the sound of a plane passing overhead.

Interestingly, mnemonists, or memory specialists, use emotion to their advantage to remember. One famous mnemonist, studied by the renowned Russian scientist Luria, experienced sensations on his skin, tasted a particular taste, and saw a particular color every time he heard a certain note of music. He consciously made each memory an intense emotional experience and, therefore, unforgettable. Unfortunately, this man became so good at remembering that he had trouble forgetting. This made it impossible for him to function well on a daily basis, until he worked out a method to actively forget.

(He needed to write down each memory he needed to forget on a blackboard and erase it!) Thus we can see the value of forgetting.

THE BOTTOM LINE

The human brain is an ever-changing, ever-evolving organ that has the capability to acquire and retain new information when it is well into its eighth or ninth decade. It is also the organ of memory, that hard-to-define concept that we depend on every second of every day. What happens when that "friend" begins to slip away from us, not just infrequently but on a daily basis? Could it be something serious? Could it be Alzheimer's disease?

Chapter 2

Could It Be Alzheimer's Disease?

In today's society, when an older person experiences memory lapses, the first thing that often pops into the minds of the person and those around that individual is "Alzheimer's disease." Yet there are a number of conditions that can explain these everyday lapses. Furthermore, it is very difficult for an individual, and often even for nonspecialized medical professionals, to tell the difference between these conditions.

Here are five real patients I have seen in my practice. Write down what you think might be the cause of their memory difficulties. The answers come up later in the chapter.

Susan is a seventy-four-year-old housewife with a history of heart problems. Her husband died two years ago and she became very depressed. Her doctor prescribed antidepressants, and although she initially responded, over the last several months she has become progressively more forgetful. A doting grandmother, she forgot her granddaughter's birthday. She lives alone and has stopped taking care of the bills. Her son, who lives about a hundred miles away, visited her at home to find her disheveled and unwashed. Though she was always a meticulous housekeeper, her kitchen was overflowing with dishes. She seemed confused, and she didn't know what day it was.

Mary is a fifty-six-year-old woman who has experienced memory loss over the past four years. She has trouble remembering her appointments, cannot remember what movie she saw yesterday, and frequently loses the lists she makes to keep her from forgetting what she needs to do. At her job as an assistant manager at a bank, she has trouble remembering what was discussed at meetings and conferences, and she is afraid she will make mistakes. She forgets words and has lost her wallet twice in the last month. She has also become more irritable in general and tends to snap at the slightest trigger.

All of these symptoms have Mary so concerned that she is now having trouble sleeping, which is only adding to her stress level. So far she feels she has been able to hide much of her forgetfulness, but she fears a day may soon come when she will not be able to do so any longer and will lose her job.

George is sixty-two, an engineer for the railroad. He has noticed that lately he has had trouble remembering names, something he always prided himself on. He has had to rely on lists to remember things. His company changed over to a new computer system and he seemed to have more trouble learning the system than he thought he should. His family made little jokes now about his "old-timer's" disease, and he was secretly worried that he had Alzheimer's. He began to notice progressively more difficulty with his memory, and finally, after not being able to locate his car in a large supermarket parking lot one afternoon, he panicked. That's when he showed up at my office for an evaluation in secret, without his family's knowledge.

* * *

Beatrice is a gregarious seventy-one-year-old woman who helps her husband in his plumbing business. She is the office manager and jane of all trades, handling emergencies and routine matters all at the same time. She has also managed to raise four kids and still baby-sits her numerous grandchildren in her spare time. Over the last two years, she has had some trouble with her memory, which has made it more difficult to multitask. She has cut down on the number of days at the office and has hired a part-timer to fill in the gap. She says she is not depressed and enjoys relaxing on the front stoop as much as the next person.

Allen is a sixty-eight-year-old professor at an Ivy League university. He is fluent in three languages and travels the world writing books. Throughout his career, Allen has been admired for his sharp wit and outgoing personality. Lately, however, he has been concerned about his memory and feels like his mind has slowed down. His wife of forty years, also a professor, says that he seems fine, although he forgets names and dates occasionally. She feels he is making too much of nothing. "Who doesn't forget as they get older?" she asks. "He has a better memory than me!" However, Allen says he has had trouble organizing and writing his latest book. He has become depressed and worried about what might be going on. His worrying has placed a great deal of stress on his marriage, and his wife is also concerned that too much stress will cause his already high blood pressure to surge even higher.

And here is the diagnosis and treatment each of these patients received.

MEDICATIONS AND MEDICAL CONDITIONS

When Susan's son brought his mother in to see me and I did an evaluation, I quickly learned that Susan had had cardiac problems for many years and was on medications that had been prescribed to her by her cardiologist. Although the antidepressants had improved her depression, she had not been good about taking her cardiac medications and was using them improperly. Medications, especially those prescribed for heart conditions, can lead to problems with memory. I recommended that she see her cardiologist immediately, and he realized what was happening. The doctor corrected the medications, and Susan was back to her old self in no time at all.

Susan reminds me of a similar situation involving a fifty-eight-year-old registered nurse, Emma, who was brought in to see me by her daughter because Emma's memory had deteriorated over the previous year. She had had surgery for a benign brain tumor at the beginning of the year and the family had assumed that her memory loss, bedwetting, and disorientation were due to the surgery. I ran several tests and discovered that Emma had new-onset diabetes, and proper treatment soon cured her memory problems and bedwetting. I had not made a diagnosis of diabetes since the first years of my training, but it was a humbling experience.

ENDOCRINE ENCEPHALOPATHY: "I'M FIFTY-FIVE AND LOSING MY MIND"

Mary turned out to have an endocrine encephalopathy (dysfunction of the brain) related to menopause. She had undergone menopause four years previously, and although her hot flashes had resolved over the first year, her memory continued to trip her up. She felt her thinking was foggy and she "mostly felt like an idiot." She was ashamed of her irritability and tried to curb it but could not seem to help herself. I prescribed treatment with natural estrogen, and her symptoms resolved within three months.

Barbara Sherwin and colleagues at McGill University first

investigated the cognitive changes in women who underwent menopause suddenly as the result of hysterectomies. They found these women had deficits in memory, in verbal fluency, and in concentration in a pattern akin to that seen in early Alzheimer's disease. Dominique Toran-Allerand at Columbia University demonstrated that estrogen deficiency led to a loss of synapses and pruning on nerve cells in animal brains and that replacement with the hormone erased these problems.

Since then, there has been a booming interest in the field. I myself became involved in the connection between hormones and memory in a serendipitous fashion. Although today I see many women for whom hormone therapy is the answer to their memory problems, there was a time when this connection was not yet clear in my mind. At that time, a sixty-year-old woman named Bernadette came to see me. Her symptoms were so consistent with Alzheimer's disease that this was the diagnosis she was given. I prescribed Aricept (a drug that helps slow progression of the disease) as well as hormone replacement therapy, because I felt it could also help slow the disease process.

She came back to see me six months later, and she had no symptoms of Alzheimer's disease. I then stopped the Aricept, continued with the hormone replacement therapy, and to this day, more than six years later, she is mentally sharp, active in her community, and feels wonderful. Apparently her memory problems had been related to a decline in estrogen and not Alzheimer's disease. Bernadette's case was a classic example of the impact of hormones on memory loss and the importance of exploring this possibility in women in menopause who complain of memory loss.

These women are not alone. In a study I presented at the North American Menopause Society, women going through menopause were six times more likely to have memory complaints than women of the same age who were not menopausal. In this study of 225 women, 60 percent of women in their menopausal years had difficulties with memory and the ability to think clearly, and many of them had unrealistic—yet real to them—fears that they were on the road to dementia. For some women, the fear is based on what they've heard or read about Alzheimer's disease and memory loss. For others, their parents have been diagnosed with dementia and they worry that their memory lapses mean they are developing the disease. Many do not realize not only that Alzheimer's disease is just one form of dementia, but that even if they do have dementia, some forms are reversible (which I discuss later in this chapter). In addition, there are many reasons why a person might experience memory loss, which are explained in the box "Causes of Memory Loss."

But quite often, the only "problem" these women have is that they are experiencing memory difficulties because of a dramatic decline in their estrogen levels, as well as a brain chemical called acetylcholine—two natural events that occur with menopause. Estrogen improves blood flow to the brain and stimulates the growth of neurons. It also enhances the activity of acetylcholine, which plays a critical role in learning. Therefore, low levels of estrogen often spell memory problems.

The role of estrogen and menopause in memory is a fascinating topic. We explore the relationship in more detail in chapters 5 and 8.

Causes of Memory Loss

- Aging: Some memory loss occurs naturally with age. Termed "age-associated memory loss," it typically includes forgetting of names, dates, and other details, but it does not significantly impact daily functioning.
- Medications: Some medications can cause memory problems; among them are barbiturates, benzodi-

azepines, blood pressure medications, heart medications, and muscle relaxants. Talk to your doctor about medications you or your loved one are taking.

- Depression: Common symptoms of depression include problems with memory, thinking clearly, and concentration.
- Alcoholism and drugs: Heavy consumption of alcohol causes brain cell death and memory loss. Also drugs such as methamphetamines can cause permanent memory loss.
- Medical conditions such as seizures and sepsis, uremia, and liver failure.
- Head trauma: Injuries to the head from a fall, traffic accident, physical assault, or sports injury may cause memory problems, difficulty with speech and language, and changes in personality.
- Stroke: Stroke is a very common cause of memory loss.
- Endocrine encephalopathy: Memory problems related to estrogen, thyroid, or other hormone deficiencies include trouble finding the right words and difficulty with concentration.
- Brain infections: These conditions, including HIV, herpes, and meningitis, damage neurons, which in turn can affect memory.
- Chronic autoimmune conditions such as multiple sclerosis and lupus cause memory loss by damaging brain networks.
- Brain tumors cause memory loss by either compressing or destroying neurons.
- Alzheimer's disease: The most common type of dementia, it is characterized by progressive memory loss.
- Other neurodegenerative conditions: In addition to Alzheimer's disease, other neurodegenerative conditions (in

which the nerve cells are damaged) include Lewy body dementia, Parkinson's disease, and Pick's disease, among others.

AGE-ASSOCIATED MEMORY IMPAIRMENT

After George underwent testing, I determined that he had age-associated memory impairment; that is, the extent of his memory loss was considered to be normal for a person his age and merely a natural part of the aging process. He was greatly relieved by the diagnosis and called back a month later to say his memory was great, although I had not prescribed any medication. It turned out that a good evaluation and education about his symptoms was all the treatment he required.

George nicely illustrates the principle of what happens when we look at the world through what I call "the-fear-of-Alzheimer's-disease-tinted glasses." Small lapses in memory, common to all of us, assume an ominous meaning, signaling a condition that almost always pales in comparison with the actual one. Imagination is no match for reality. Once reassured, George was able to revert to his usual functioning. I find that patients with age-associated memory impairment have trouble with naming and more difficulty with learning new tasks, but this does not interfere with their daily functioning.

In addition, stress is an important contributor to memory, as it affects both memory functioning and mood. Perhaps best known as the stress hormone, cortisol is released at high levels by the adrenal glands in response to stress. Experts already know that high cortisol levels have a negative effect on memory, even in healthy adults. In fact, chronically high levels of this hormone can damage the hippocampus, the area of the brain where memory (especially short-term memory) and emotions are controlled. These facts have led some researchers to suggest that stress is a significant factor in memory loss among older adults.

MILD COGNITIVE IMPAIRMENT

Unlike George, whose memory challenges are age-related, Beatrice has mild cognitive impairment. This lies somewhere in between normal memory lapses associated with aging and more definitive signs of progressive memory loss associated with dementias. Basically, individuals in this category have no trouble with activities of daily living—dressing, eating, shopping, household chores—and maintain good reasoning and thinking abilities, but they experience a decline in short-term memory that is worse than that usually seen in people their age. This decline appears to be faster than that associated with normal aging, but slower than the memory loss in people who have Alzheimer's disease. Most have some difficulty with functioning, but not of sufficient severity to be labeled Alzheimer's.

The number of people with mild cognitive impairment is not known. Some studies are being done to determine its prevalence, but it may be some time before we have reliable figures, given that different doctors use varying criteria to make a diagnosis. There are, however, some guidelines doctors can follow.

Signs of Mild Cognitive Impairment

Only a doctor can make an accurate diagnosis of mild cognitive impairment, using a series of screening and diagnostic tools (see chapter 4). However, you can help your physician with that task if you note any of the following symptoms.

This list is a guideline only. Do not jump to any conclusions if some or many of these symptoms apply to you or a loved one.

- Episodes of forgetfulness
- Increased need to rely on written reminders for appointments, shopping items, dates (birthdays, anniversaries, etc.), or other daily activities
- Difficulty retaining information read in newspapers, magazines, or books
- More trouble than usual remembering the names of friends or acquaintances
- Increased difficulty finding the right word when speaking
- Tendency to misplace or lose items

If you're like most people, you've had occasions when you were speaking and suddenly couldn't find the "right" word. You may have said, "It's on the tip of my tongue." Then, perhaps within seconds or minutes, you "found" the word, and you continued your conversation. Marilyn Albert, a neuropsychologist at Harvard University, calls this "lost-and-found" experience the "aha! phenomenon." She notes that individuals who have normal memory lapses typically recall the word, while people who have mild cognitive impairment or a more serious type of memory problem usually don't experience this phenomenon.

Mild Cognitive Impairment and Alzheimer's Disease

A question I often hear is, "Does having mild cognitive impairment mean I'm at greater risk of getting Alzheimer's disease?" Over time, more than half the people with a diagnosis of mild cognitive impairment go on to develop Alzheimer's within four years of their initial diagnosis, but the rest get better, and some stay unchanged.

It is my belief that patients with mild cognitive impairment should be treated and followed over time with serial testing of different abilities, including language, writing, reading, reasoning, and understanding. Such testing should be done annually. A significant decline in one or more of these areas may indicate that a memory problem has progressed from mild cognitive impairment to Alzheimer's disease. However, adequate treatment may delay or even prevent the development of an irreversible condition such as Alzheimer's disease. The preventive measures discussed in this book in chapter 5, and especially the brain boosters in chapter 6, are ways to help retain memory and cognitive functioning.

In April 2003, researchers reported on the results of a study of donepezil (Aricept) given to 269 people with mild cognitive impairment. Donepezil is the most commonly prescribed medication for Alzheimer's disease (see chapter 7), but its benefits in people who have mild cognitive impairment are not known. This study found that six months of treatment with donepezil caused a "very modest" improvement in cognitive functioning compared with people who took a placebo (sugar pill). Clearly more research is needed.

ALZHEIMER'S DISEASE

Did you pick Allen as the person with Alzheimer's disease? How did you make the right diagnosis? In fact, Allen had been to two other doctors and had been dismissed as not having a problem. He tested with an IQ of 142 (which is higher than more than 99 percent of the population), but in some types of memory his scores plummeted very low. He had Alzheimer's disease, a neurodegenerative (destruction of neurons in the brain) disease that primarily affects people who are sixty-five years or older. This type is known as late-onset Alzheimer's. A much rarer form, known as early-onset Alzheimer's, affects less than 5 percent of those who get the disease, and can in very rare instances appear in individuals as young as twenty-four.

Dementia is a general term for a condition in which a person loses memory and other mental abilities of sufficient severity to interfere with functioning. Alzheimer's is one of many types of dementia, and by far the most common, with the next being vascular dementia. By the age of eighty-five, one of three people will suffer with dementia. A common feature for all types of dementia is the death of nerve cells in the brain.

Various changes occur in the brain of people who have Alzheimer's disease, and it's these changes—as well as those that researchers may not have yet discovered—that can help them learn more about diagnosing, preventing, and treating the disease. We talk about some of those changes here, as they will help you better understand the cognitive and personality changes that may be occurring with your loved one.

What Is Alzheimer's Disease?

Alzheimer's disease is characterized by the dying of cells in the brain. The first place this destruction usually takes place is in the hippocampus, which, as you'll recall, plays a major role in short-term memory. The hippocampus is like the main gate to the City of Stored Memory. This gate is important for directing memory to various areas to be stored and then used to retrieve memories.

In Alzheimer's disease, cell death occurs when toxic substances are deposited in the brain, a process that begins decades before the onset of any symptoms. In fact, the earliest changes in the brain occur in persons in their thirties.

From the hippocampus the cell damage typically spreads to the cerebral cortex (frontal, parietal, and temporal lobes; see Figure 1 in chapter 1). Damage to these areas affects emotions and instincts, as well as the ability to communicate, make decisions, and perform simple tasks.

Neurotransmitters—the brain's messengers—are also affected in Alzheimer's disease. It's important to know a little about each of these substances, because some of the medications and complementary remedies we discuss later (chapters 7 and 8) have an effect on them. The levels of all of the following neurotransmitters typically decline in people who have Alzheimer's disease:

- Acetylcholine: involved with the creation and recall of memories; also learning and attention
- Dopamine: plays a major role in physical movement and in mood and psychosis
- Glutamate: involved with long-term memory and learning
- Norepinephrine: affects emotions
- Serotonin: has a major role in depression, anxiety, and mood

As the disease progresses over time, more and more neurons are destroyed in more areas of the brain, more synapses are lost, neurotransmitter levels continue to decline, and the brain shrinks. This process proceeds at a different pace in each individual. Once the first signs of the disease appear, the course for Alzheimer's is typically two to twenty years (average, eight to ten years).

The Mystery of Tangles and Plaques

Tangles and plaques are names given to the changes that occur in the brains of people who have Alzheimer's disease. Your doctor may mention these substances, as they appear to play a very significant role in the disease. In fact, some of the treatments for Alzheimer's focus on eliminating tangles and plaques, as you'll learn in chapters 7 and 8.

Tangles are twisted threads of the abnormal form of a protein called "tau," which when healthy helps to maintain the shape of nerve cells and to transport materials within them. In illnesses like Alzheimer's, the abnormal form of tau clumps like a tangle of hair within nerve cells, eventually causing them to die.

In addition, outside of the nerve cells, plaques made of a protein called beta-amyloid build up, which in a healthy state are excreted from the body without accumulating. These accumulations of beta-amyloid plaques outside the cells act as toxins, damaging the cells and causing them to die. Thus, both tau and beta-amyloid are found in healthy brains, but for reasons not yet understood, in illnesses like Alzheimer's disease both of these proteins undergo abnormal changes and then accumulate and ultimately harm the nerve cells.

Questions about tangles and plaques are like those of the chicken-or-the-egg debate: which comes first? Experts don't know whether tangles and plaques cause Alzheimer's disease or whether they appear as a result of the disease process, but there are fervent supporters in each camp, dubbed the "tau"ists and the "B-ap"tists (beta-amyloid protein).

Inflammation

Along with the tangles and plaques in the brains of people who have Alzheimer's disease, scientists have also found inflammation. Inflammation is one way the body works to heal itself. We usually associate it with an injury or an infection: if you cut your finger, you'll notice some swelling around the wound, or if you get an ear infection, some swelling is typically involved. Inflammation is a key symptom in arthritis, and experts have also linked inflammation in blood vessels with heart disease.

Why does inflammation occur in Alzheimer's disease? One theory is that it is the body's attempt to fight back against the accumulation or the "invasion" of plaques, which the body perceives as foreign material. In other words, certain immune cells called microglia may be trying to destroy the plaques, and in the process they trigger inflammation. It's also possible that the microglia stimulate other substances in the body that cause inflammation, including prostaglandins, C-reactive protein, and the enzyme COX-2 (cyclooxygenase). Yet another theory is that the inflammation could be the body's response to some yet unknown reaction or activity.

One recent study (*Neurology,* July 2003) of inflammation and Alzheimer's disease in more than 3,000 people found that individuals who had the highest levels of inflammatory substances in their blood (substances such as interleukin-6 and C-reactive protein) had more memory problems and cognitive decline than those with low levels of these substances. While investigators try to uncover the mystery of inflammation in Alzheimer's disease, they know that some studies show that taking anti-inflammatory medications appears to help many people who have the disease. This information will hopefully prove helpful in finding more effective treatments for Alzheimer's disease. However, a recent study found no benefit from the use of anti-inflammatory agents in Alzheimer's. You can read more about the possible benefits and risks of anti-inflammatory drugs in Alzheimer's disease in chapter 7.

Calcium

We often think of calcium as something that's good for bone health, but it also plays a role in helping messages pass between nerve cells. Research indicates that accumulation of beta-amyloid plaque may cause calcium to enter neurons in excessive amounts and thus cause brain cells to die. **This doesn't mean, however, that you should reduce your consumption of calcium or calcium-containing foods as a way to prevent Alzheimer's disease.** The fact that beta-amyloid plaque has this effect on calcium is not related to your intake of this essential mineral.

Oxidative Stress

Once again, accumulation of beta-amyloid plaque may cause even more problems in the brain: it can damage mitochondria, cell structures that produce energy for the cells. When mitochondria malfunction, they produce an overabundance of molecules called free radicals, which causes a process called oxidative stress. One result of oxidative stress is cell destruction. Experts have known for many years that oxidative stress plays a key role in heart disease and cancer. Now there is evidence that it is also a major player in Alzheimer's disease.

Oxidative stress will come up again when we talk about prevention and treatment of Alzheimer's disease, as there are ways you can reduce this type of damage (see chapters 5 and 8).

SIGNS AND SYMPTOMS OF ALZHEIMER'S DISEASE

Now we get to the signs and symptoms of Alzheimer's disease. I would first like to stress that in most individuals, Alzheimer's disease progresses very slowly. Thus, if we can slow progression by even two or three years, or delay onset by that amount of time, we would accomplish a great deal toward maintaining people's independent functioning until death. Second, in the early stages of an illness like Alzheimer's, the condition may only be apparent to the sufferer and possibly a few others. He or she may be able to function in complex jobs without difficulty. For example, I have several patients who, with my encouragement, continue to function in their jobs despite mild Alzheimer's disease.

Finally, I want to address the question of stages. There is nothing I dislike more than having to "stage" a condition like Alzheimer's disease. In illnesses such as cancer, accurate staging is based on pathological changes in or at lymph nodes, spread of the disease to other organs, and so on. These changes are relatively easy to see and document, and they predict response to treatment and prognosis. Primarily clinical chronic illnesses like diabetes or hypertension rarely get "staged" in a clinical setting. However, patients and families often feel the need to have a stage attributed to Alzheimer's disease. They ask, "What stage do you think my husband is in?" or "How long do you think it will be before my wife gets to stage two (or three or four)?"

In my opinion, this arbitrary staging, based on clinical symptoms, without any relation to the person's prior level of functioning, has little clinical use. Instead, I try to answer the question that I believe families and patients are really asking: *"How long can I continue to live a productive life?"* In this instance, I try to get both the patient and the family to give me their best estimate as to when they believe symptoms first occurred. This allows me to plot a course that will predict future performance.

There are certain indicators of good prognosis in Alzheimer's, and indicators of poor prognosis. Here are some of the main ones I consider.

Good Prognosis	**Poor Prognosis**
Good function prior to dementia onset	Strokes
High education	Early language difficulties
Physically fit	Early hallucinations or agitation
No language deficits	Difficulties with ambulation
Supportive family	Rapid early progression
Good vocabulary	Cardiac disease, poorly controlled blood pressure

With treatment, I have many patients who have continued to stay at current levels of functioning for up to seven years. I think Alzheimer's disease should be viewed like any other chronic, potentially devastating illness like, say, hypertension. Some hypertensive patients may go on to develop strokes and paralysis or malignant hypertension and die from it, but most people with hypertension are able to live productive, functional lives if they follow the right medication management. Hypertension is not curable, but early diagnosis is important for future prognosis. So too with Alzheimer's disease.

Allen Has Mild Alzheimer's Disease

This earliest stage of Alzheimer's disease can be difficult to detect, as the signs and symptoms are often very subtle (see box, "Some Early Warning Signs of Alzheimer's Disease").

Depression is often a presenting symptom of Alzheimer's disease, even before any problems with memory become apparent. Research indicates that symptoms of depression may develop as much as three years before some people are diagnosed with Alzheimer's disease. Knowing this, it becomes apparent that recognizing and treating depression is important, especially among older adults, and that testing for Alzheimer's disease at this time may be indicated for some individuals who are at risk for the disease or who are concerned about it. In fact, major depression affects 30 to 50 percent of people who later develop Alzheimer's disease.

Some Early Warning Signs of Alzheimer's Disease

Here are some early warning signs of Alzheimer's disease. These symptoms are often similar to those of mild cognitive impairment, a precursor of Alzheimer's disease. It's important to remember that individuals may not experience all of these signs, and while forgetfulness is often the first warning sign, it must persist for months and grow progressively worse to be considered a symptom of Alzheimer's disease.

- Failure to remember recent events
- Avoidance of new people and/or places
- Difficulty with abstract ideas or thoughts, such as math
- Losing one's place in a conversation, or having difficulty completing sentences or finding the right words
- Decline of interest in one's surroundings
- Reduced desire to take initiative, meet new people, take a vacation, or start new projects
- Problems with concentration and/or comprehension.

Many people realize this is happening to them and so they try to hide it.

- Noticeable loss of interest in appearance or social courtesies; individuals who were once conscientious about their clothing or housekeeping skills become unkempt or sloppy.
- Depression

Although the symptoms listed in the box are typically the first outward indications that someone has Alzheimer's disease, changes in the brain begin years before these signs become obvious. Early detection of these changes in the brain are possible (see chapter 4, "Uncovering Alzheimer's Disease"). In fact, people who are at high risk of developing Alzheimer's disease because of a genetic predisposition can undergo testing for early detection. This is a controversial issue, and is discussed in chapter 3.

Some of the men and women who came to me who are in the early stage of Alzheimer's disease are still working full- or part-time; others are retired, engaged in volunteer activities, or travel; they are still socializing with family and friends and trying to go about life as usual. But often they are also harboring fear, anger, uncertainty, and a feeling of helplessness. These emotions create stress for the individual and for his or her loved ones, and tend to make the episodes of forgetfulness and other memory problems worse.

Harold, a seventy-two-year-old retired engineer, and his wife, Cynthia, a seventy-four-year-old retired nurse, are dealing with emotional issues that have arisen as Cynthia's memory declines. They were always active in their younger years, and they were both in the full swing of their retirement years—traveling to Europe and China, visiting friends around the

United States, volunteering at a local children's shelter—when they got Cynthia's diagnosis. I encouraged them to continue their activities, as both the physical and mental stimulation were great medicine for Cynthia. They were both grateful for that advice and agreed to follow it.

Harold admits, however, that sometimes he finds Cynthia sitting alone in her room, crying. "At first she was angry," he says, "and then over time her tears were more from sadness and a feeling of helplessness. She keeps saying, 'What happens when I don't even know my grandchildren anymore?' All I can say is that that day may never come, that we must concentrate on the good times that we have right now. But it makes me sad too, and angry, and sometimes I don't know what to do with that anger." Fortunately, there are ways—medically, naturally, and psychologically—patients and their families can help alleviate and deal with these symptoms and feelings. I talk about them in chapters 7, 8, 9, and 10.

OTHER TYPES OF DEMENTIA

Although Alzheimer's disease makes up about 60 to 65 percent of all cases of dementia, the remaining 35 to 40 percent can be attributed to approximately fifty different causes, many of which are rare. It's important to remember that although Alzheimer's disease is not reversible, a few other types of dementia are. These, along with common types of irreversible dementia, are discussed here. It is also possible for any of these other types of dementia to occur along with Alzheimer's disease.

Vascular Dementia

Approximately 15 percent of people who have dementia have Alzheimer's disease along with vascular dementia. This irreversible type of dementia can occur when the flow of blood to the brain is interrupted, causing strokes. People who have vascular dementia may experience symptoms of stroke such as weakness or paralysis on one side of the body, difficulty with speech, and vision problems, but many patients have no such symptoms ("silent strokes"). Vascular dementia can be distinguished from Alzheimer's disease with the use of imaging techniques like the MRI (magnetic resonance imaging) and a careful history and examination.

Frontal Lobe Dementia

The front of the brain is occupied by the frontal lobe, and a number of forms of dementia are associated with damage in this area. One of the more common forms of frontal lobe dementia is Pick's disease, which is characterized by dramatic personality changes, including aggression, rudeness, inappropriate behavior in public, and lack of inhibition. Other symptoms include loss of short-term memory, impaired speech, and a lack of initiative.

Frontal lobe dementia is irreversible. It can affect people of any age, but it usually appears between the ages of forty and sixty-five. About 50 percent of people with frontal lobe dementia have a family history of the disease. It's estimated that up to 10 percent of patients with dementia have the frontal lobe type.

Dementia with Lewy Bodies

While Alzheimer's disease is associated with deposits of amyloid and tau proteins, another type of irreversible dementia is characterized by deposits of another protein, Lewy bodies. About 15 to 20 percent of dementias may be of this type. Lewy bodies can destroy brain cells and cause symptoms that are similar to both Alzheimer's disease and Parkinson's disease, a condition in which individuals experience tremors, problems walking, speech difficulties, and stiff limbs.

Patients with Lewy body–related dementia suffer from frequent falls, Parkinsonian features, early onset of hallucinations and psychiatric symptoms, and increased sensitivity to certain types of medications. The illness generally progresses more rapidly than Alzheimer's disease, but is also more responsive to treatment.

Other Causes of Dementia

Doctors should also consider other causes of dementia, based on a person's medical history, current health status, and medication use. Causes that are completely or partially reversible include chronic drug abuse, brain tumors (those that can be removed), subdural hematoma (a swelling of blood on the brain that is usually the result of trauma to the head), renal failure, hypothyroidism, chronic lung disease, and hypoglycemia (low blood sugar levels). Other types of dementia that are not reversible include AIDS dementia complex, Parkinson's disease, and that associated with Creutzfeldt-Jakob disease, a rapidly progressive disease that is characterized by dementia and muscle spasms (a form of which is popularly called Mad Cow disease).

LOOKS LIKE DEMENTIA . . . BUT IT'S NOT

Just because someone has symptoms that appear to be those of dementia doesn't automatically mean dementia is the diagnosis. Two conditions that have symptoms that mimic those of dementia—especially when they appear in older adults—are depression and delirium. Why is it important to properly diagnose those conditions? Because, unlike dementias, depression and delirium can be treated effectively and eliminated.

If you look again at some of the symptoms listed in the earlier box ("Some Early Warning Signs of Alzheimer's Disease")—decline in interest, reduced desire to take initiative, loss of concentration—these are also symptoms of depression. In fact, especially among older people, depression can have a significant impact on memory, concentration, and the ability to think clearly, symptoms not always seen in younger people who are depressed. Depression is common among older adults, largely because this time of life can be accompanied by great stressors, such as health problems, death of a spouse and/or friends and family members, retirement, loss of one's home, and a decline in hormone levels.

Physicians often overlook depression in their older patients, and this oversight can result in a misdiagnosis. Talk to your doctor about the possibility that your loved one may be experiencing symptoms of depression. It is also possible for depression to occur along with dementia.

Delirium is a condition characterized by disorientation, confused speech, agitation, hallucinations, and an alteration of consciousness. One telltale indication that someone is experiencing delirium and not dementia is that the symptoms of delirium come on suddenly rather than over time. Delirium is frequently seen in older adults who have serious health problems, including heart disease, urinary tract or other infections, malnutrition, or lung disease. It can also be a side effect of taking one or more medications, which is a common practice among older adults.

Dementia	**Delirium**
Slow, progressive onset over months to years	Abrupt onset, usually days or weeks
Attention generally not affected	Very short attention span
Normal consciousness level	Consciousness affected, may fluctuate
Hallucinations may appear late in disease	Hallucinations, especially visual and tactile, are common
Agitation and aggression late in course of disease	Agitation common early; often occurs in setting of medical crises
Normal speech	Slurred speech
Short-term memory poor first; long-term good until late in the disease	Short- and long-term memory poor

THE BOTTOM LINE

Memory loss is not a sure sign of Alzheimer's disease; in fact, in many cases, what you or a loved one may be experiencing is a reversible condition, such as memory loss caused by a hormone deficiency, medication use, or a medical condition. Memory loss may also be attributed to mild cognitive impairment or to a type of dementia besides Alzheimer's. The treatment approach for each type of memory loss situation is different, which is why it's so crucial to pay close attention to the signs and symptoms you or a loved one is experiencing and to report them as accurately as possible to your physician.

Chapter 3

Causes of and Risk Factors for Alzheimer's Disease

When Alois Alzheimer first discovered the tangles and plaques that are the trademark of the disease that bears his name, he would probably never have thought that nearly one hundred years later, scientists and physicians would still be puzzled about what exactly triggers this form of dementia. Not that experts don't have many candidates in the ring: advanced age, genetics, Down syndrome, history of head trauma, family history, environmental toxins, ethnicity, gender, stress, low educational status, and alcohol are among the possible risk factors—or causes—being investigated by researchers around the world.

To this list I add factors not typically considered by most physicians: early menopause and hysterectomy in my female patients. This is a topic I have mentioned before and will talk about again, because it is so important for women to consider if they are having memory problems.

Based on years of clinical evidence, I believe that more risk factors must be considered, including high-cholesterol, high-fat diet; obesity; diabetes; hypertension; sedentary lifestyle; and high homocysteine levels. If this list looks familiar, that's because these items are risk factors for stroke. In fact, all the risk factors for stroke and heart disease are also risk factors for Alzheimer's disease.

Increasing scientific evidence links these three major health problems. A study published in the *New England Journal of Medicine* in March 2003 provided strong evidence linking stroke, Alzheimer's disease, and narrowed blood vessels in the brain. The Alzheimer's Association agrees that "there is a growing body of evidence identifying known risk factors for heart disease, including high blood pressure and high cholesterol, as risk factors for Alzheimer's." The good news about symptoms like high blood pressure and high cholesterol is that they are preventable and controllable, which means people can take steps to help prevent the serious diseases that go along with them—including Alzheimer's disease. I discuss preventive measures in chapter 5.

Generally, scientists believe that Alzheimer's disease is caused by a combination of genetics and other factors, and that the formula that triggers the disease is different for each person. In this chapter we look at the possible and probable causes of Alzheimer's disease. One reason it is important to understand these factors is that for many of them, their opposites are actually *preventive* measures (for example, lack of physical activity may be a risk factor, while regular exercise may help prevent Alzheimer's).

Notice I say "may help prevent" Alzheimer's disease. Thus far we do not have a cure for Alzheimer's disease, and no one is absolutely certain what causes it. We do, however, have research that shows many different factors that clearly contribute to or are associated with it. For now, taking preventive steps is your best bet to avoid Alzheimer's disease.

Another topic to explore in this chapter is a controversial one: whether individuals who are at known or perceived high risk for the disease should undergo genetic testing, and the impact of such a decision on the individual tested and his or her family. A decision to pursue genetic testing is a highly personal one, and I hope I can help those who are considering this option.

ADVANCED AGE

One of the few things researchers do know is that the chance of getting Alzheimer's disease increases as we age. That risk doubles about every five years after age sixty-five: of people ages sixty-five to seventy-four, 3 percent will be diagnosed with Alzheimer's disease; between seventy-five and eighty-four, the number is 19 percent; among those eighty-five years and older, the incidence is approximately 47 percent.

These figures clearly show that the majority of older people don't get Alzheimer's disease, which means it is *not* an inevitable part of aging. Other factors must be involved.

GENETICS AND FAMILY HISTORY

Sometimes people come to me full of fear because one of their parents had Alzheimer's disease, or their sibling has the disease, and now they are experiencing some lapses in memory and they want to know, "Do I have the disease, too?" We know that approximately 30 percent of all people who have Alzheimer's disease have a family history of dementia. But that's only contributing 30 percent to the cause; what about the other 70 percent? Clearly, genetics and family history are not the only factors. In a very large study with more than 5,000 parents and siblings that I conducted along with colleagues at Columbia University, we found that the lifetime risk for developing Alzheimer's was 26 percent in those who had a family history and 19 percent in those who did not. So while there is an increased risk of Alzheimer's disease in children of patients with the condition, it is not a very large one.

Early-Onset Alzheimer's Disease

There is a rare exception to this statement. Early-onset Alzheimer's disease, usually defined as onset of the disease before the age of sixty, is caused by genetic mutations to three different chromosomes, numbers 1, 14, and 21. The mutation may be passed down over the generations and can cause the disease to occur in people as young as twenty-four. Approximately 200,000 people in the United States (or 5 percent of the 4 million who have Alzheimer's disease) have early-onset disease.

Familial (multiple family members with the disease) early-onset Alzheimer's disease is strongly hereditary. Nearly everyone who has any of the three forms of the mutated genes develops the disease. Each child who has a parent with a mutated gene has a 50 percent chance of inheriting the form that causes Alzheimer's disease. The mutations can be detected in some families using a special testing procedure. Use of this test raises many sensitive ethical and legal issues, because at this point in time, we cannot prevent or cure early-onset Alzheimer's disease. For a discussion of this controversy, see the box "The Right to Know?"

Genes and Late-Onset Disease

So far, scientists have identified a form of one gene that is a major risk factor for late-onset Alzheimer's. Known as apolipoprotein, or ApoE, it comes in three forms, or alleles—

ApoE2, ApoE3, and ApoE4—and is found on chromosome #19. One of these forms is inherited from each parent. Of the three, ApoE4 causes a greater amount of beta-amyloid to accumulate in the brain, but exactly why the ApoE4 gene makes this happen is not understood.

Every individual inherits two copies of the ApoE gene, and the forms may be the same as each other or different. People who inherit the ApoE4 gene have a greater risk of developing late-onset Alzheimer's disease than those who have either of the other two types, but having this gene *does not mean you will definitely get Alzheimer's.* Thus, while having the gene increases people's susceptibility for the disease, it's certainly not a guarantee they will get it. In fact, in the general population:

- About 60 percent of people inherit two ApoE3 genes, which does not increase their risk of developing Alzheimer's. This means about 50 percent of this group will develop the disease by about age eighty to eighty-five.
- About 25 percent of people inherit one copy of ApoE4, which increases their risk of developing Alzheimer's disease by up to four times.
- About 2 percent inherit two copies of ApoE4, which increases their risk of getting Alzheimer's disease by about ten times, but it still is not a guarantee the disease will develop.
- About 16 percent of people inherit the ApoE2 gene. Individuals who have one ApoE2 gene and one ApoE3 gene (11 percent of the population) are partially protected from Alzheimer's disease, as they have to live into their late nineties before their risk of getting the disease is 50 percent of normal. Only 0.5 percent of people inherit two copies of the ApoE2 gene, and they have the least risk of getting Alzheimer's disease.

The presence of Down syndrome is another type of genetic risk factor for Alzheimer's. Nearly all people with Down syndrome who reach forty years or older show changes in their brains that are consistent with Alzheimer's disease.

The Right to Know?

Do people have the right to know if they have the genetic makeup that puts them at high risk for developing Alzheimer's disease? Generally, the answer is yes. But I believe there are several factors individuals should take into consideration before they decide to undergo genetic testing.

One is the fact that genetic testing for the most common type of Alzheimer's disease—late-onset disease—is far from conclusive, as we have already explained (see "Genes and Late-Onset Disease"). Thus I almost never use genetic testing for late-onset Alzheimer's disease, except on the rare occasion when it will aid in the diagnosis. Yet there are some people who insist on being tested. However, these individuals need to realize that the information they get is often of little or no clinical use, and can be detrimental. Once this information becomes part of their medical records, there is the possibility that an insurance company that discovers that someone has the ApoE4 gene may choose not to cover them for long-term insurance or other insurance benefits.

Testing for familial early-onset Alzheimer's disease, however, can be a different story. Many people who have early-onset Alzheimer's disease are referred to me, and so the questions of whether other family members should undergo genetic testing often arise. One lovely family I now treat illustrates the situation.

In the late 1950s, Marie and her husband, Robert, met

and married while they were still in their late teens. They both loved children, and they had three lovely children over a span of five years. Soon after the birth of their third child, Robert began to experience increasingly severe problems with dementia. By age thirty-five he was confined to a nursing home, and Marie was left to raise her children on her own.

When her oldest son, Mark, was twenty-eight, he became depressed and was having trouble at work. Mark and his wife came to see me ten years ago, without a diagnosis. After an extensive examination, I diagnosed him as having Alzheimer's, which was devastating to them both. Unlike late-onset Alzheimer's, early-onset Alzheimer's can be very aggressive. Then the second son also became ill. The question then was: did the daughter, the youngest, have the disease as well? I, along with colleagues in the United States and Canada, was able to isolate a new gene for Alzheimer's in this family. We then tested her, and in one of the most gratifying moments of my career, I was able to give her the good news that she did not carry this gene mutation for early-onset Alzheimer's.

But the story continues, because Mark, the oldest son, has four children in their early teens. Should these children be tested for the presence of a gene mutation like the one that has left their father incapacitated? I believe we should offer these children the opportunity to undergo genetic testing, but only when they reach the age of consent. Then they can be presented with all we know (which by then will be considerably more than we know now) about early-onset Alzheimer's disease and their options, which include treatment. At the present time, treatment of early-onset Alzheimer's disease is similar to that for late-onset disease, and is aimed at trying to slow the progression of the disease and improve the quality of life of the affected individual. (All identifying features were altered for privacy protection.)

GENDER

Like genetics and family history, there are other factors over which we have no control. One fact about Alzheimer's disease that continues to puzzle experts is why more women than men develop the condition. Two factors appear to contribute to this phenomenon: women live longer than men, and so they are more likely to get the disease; and women experience a dramatic decline in estrogen levels at menopause, an event that is associated with memory loss. But are these the only possible reasons for the difference? We simply don't know.

HISTORY OF HEAD TRAUMA

Whether the history of head injury is a cause of Alzheimer's disease is uncertain. Some studies suggest that head trauma that results in a loss of consciousness is a definite risk factor for developing Alzheimer's disease. People who expose themselves to repeated head trauma, such as boxers and football players, are believed to be at high risk for the disease. Many boxers, in particular, exhibit problems with memory, concentration, speech, and other brain functions later in life.

It may be that chronic injuries, such as those suffered by boxers and some athletes, are critical factors, while the fall you took as a child from a swing that left you unconscious for a few minutes has little or no impact on whether you ever get Alzheimer's. The significance of head trauma as a risk factor is still under investigation.

LIFESTYLE: DIET AND EXERCISE

Most of the same risk factors for stroke and coronary artery disease, which include lack of physical activity, high cholesterol levels, and eating a high-fat diet, also increase the risk of developing Alzheimer's disease. One reason for this finding, published in a February 2001 article in the *Journal of the American Medical Association,* could be associated with the fact that people who have cardiovascular conditions are more likely to experience transient ischemic attacks (TIAs), which disrupt blood flow to the brain and thus negatively affect memory and other brain functions. Other studies suggest that high calorie and fat consumption can promote inflammation, which is a characteristic of the brain of people who have Alzheimer's disease (see chapter 2), as well as those who have heart disease. That's why in chapter 5, "A Pound of Prevention," I offer you some guidelines on healthy eating to help prevent Alzheimer's disease.

Dietary Fat and Alzheimer's Risk

There is much evidence that links a high-fat diet and heart disease. Many experts believe that a similar case can be made for Alzheimer's disease, given that the other risk factors for each of these serious conditions are the same. A recent study published in the *Archives of Neurology* (February 2003) suggested that people who consume a diet that is high in trans fats (hydrogenated and partially hydrogenated oils and shortening, which are found in margarines and many processed foods including baked goods, snack foods [potato chips, corn chips, popcorn], cereals, salad dressings, peanut butter, fried foods, and frozen dinners) are at greater risk of developing Alzheimer's disease. That's because trans fats, like saturated fats, raise the levels of the bad cholesterol, low-density lipoprotein (LDL). Trans fats are actually believed to be more harmful than saturated fats, however, because they also lower levels of the good cholesterol—high-density lipoprotein (HDL)—and raise the levels of C-reactive protein, a substance that causes inflammation in the blood vessels.

Homocysteine

The word "homocysteine" has become more familiar for people as researchers have found that high levels of this amino acid are associated with an increased risk of stroke. Now experts are indicating that high homocysteine levels can damage blood vessels in the brain, which in turn can result in dementia. A study published in the *New England Journal of Medicine* in February 2002 reported that the risk of dementia increased as homocysteine levels rose. In fact, people with high levels were nearly twice as likely to develop Alzheimer's disease as individuals with low levels.

How is homocysteine related to diet? Homocysteine is normally changed into other amino acids for use by the body. However, this transformation requires lots of help from various B vitamins, especially folate (folic acid), which is found in abundance in green leafy vegetables, other vegetables, and fruit. Thus, people whose diets are low in fruits and vegetables are more likely to have high levels of homocysteine. Your doctor can administer a simple blood test to identify your levels. In chapter 5 I discuss some ways you can lower your homocysteine levels.

Exercise

When it comes to exercise, research suggests that people who are not physically active between the ages of twenty and fifty-nine are more likely to develop Alzheimer's disease than those who exercise regularly. The importance of this risk factor requires further investigation (see chapter 5, "A Pound of Prevention").

HISTORY OF STROKE AND CARDIOVASCULAR DISEASE

A history of stroke or cardiovascular disease, or the presence of risk factors for these diseases (e.g., high blood pressure, obesity, diabetes, smoking, high cholesterol), is a major risk factor for Alzheimer's disease. In 2002, a University of Pittsburgh School of Medicine study found that people who have cardiovascular disease—angina, heart attack, peripheral vascular disease—have a 30 percent increased risk of dementia. Because cardiovascular disease is largely preventable, this study offers good news for people who want to take preventive measures against Alzheimer's disease (see chapter 5, "A Pound of Prevention," for tips).

EARLY MENOPAUSE AND HYSTERECTOMY

As we discussed in chapter 2, most doctors don't associate a dramatic decline in estrogen levels with memory loss, but it is a relationship that deserves our attention, because the correlation is strong. Thus a few of the first questions I ask my female patients is whether they underwent early menopause (before age fifty) or if they've had a hysterectomy, as both of these situations mean their estrogen levels declined dramatically earlier in their lives. If women answer yes to either question, I also inquire if they've been taking hormone replacement therapy.

Although the research is not conclusive, there is strong evidence that estrogen helps protect against the development of Alzheimer's disease. Thus women who lose that possible protective edge early—through early menopause and/or hysterectomy—and who don't take estrogen replacement after the fact may be at higher risk of the disease.

SMOKING

A study of the effect of smoking on the development of Alzheimer's disease was done in more than 6,800 men and women aged fifty-five years or older. Compared with nonsmokers, smokers were twice as likely to develop the disease. These findings have been upheld by subsequent research. Yet there have been a few studies that suggest smoking may *protect* against Alzheimer's disease, likely because nicotine can improve memory. (This is *not* an argument in support of smoking!) This interesting finding has prompted scientists to look at possible ways to package the benefits of nicotine into a medication without retaining its negative effects.

STRESS

Stress contributes to the death of neurons in the hippocampus, which is the main routing station for memory. The hippocampus loses about 6 percent of its cells every ten years after the age of forty-five, so any additional loss of cells due to stress can make a significant difference in memory and cognitive abilities. Although studies have not yet measured the extent to which stress may be a risk factor for Alzheimer's disease, the negative impact of stress on blood pressure—which can lead to stroke—has been documented, and both of these medical conditions are strong risk factors for dementia (see "History of Stroke and Cardiovascular Disease," at left).

EDUCATION AND JOB STATUS

Several studies show a strong relationship between level of education and the likelihood that one will develop Alzheimer's disease. The first significant study, which looked specifically at educational status, was called the Nun Study. It involved analyzing the handwritten autobiographies of a group of nuns that they had completed themselves as they entered the convent and noting their structural complexity. The nuns had their brains examined after their deaths, and researchers found that those who had exhibited more complexity in their writing (more ideas per sentence) were much less likely to have accumulated tangles in their brains and to develop Alzheimer's than the nuns who had shown a low level of education.

Since then, other studies have looked at both education and job status and found that people with high educational and occupational achievements appear to be at lower risk for developing Alzheimer's disease. Naturally, these factors are not guarantees against getting Alzheimer's disease. Consider, for example, Winston Churchill and world-famous artist Norman Rockwell, who were both affected by the disease. Did their high level of mental activity prevent them from getting the disease sooner? It's an interesting speculation.

For now, however, the possible link between high educational status and less risk of Alzheimer's disease also supports something else we'll be discussing later in this book: brain exercises, the "use it or lose it" approach that helps prevent memory loss and maintains the best level of mental functioning—as well as quality of life—for as long as possible.

ALCOHOL

Consumption of alcohol is one activity that may be both detrimental and beneficial when it comes to Alzheimer's disease. The key, it seems, lies in how much alcohol people drink and what kind they choose.

Heavy drinking (five or more drinks every day or nearly every day for years) greatly speeds up the rate at which the brain shrinks, which directly affects memory and the ability to think. In fact, a condition known as alcoholic dementia is characterized by many of the same features of Alzheimer's disease. However, the exact role alcohol may play in Alzheimer's disease is still unclear.

ENVIRONMENTAL TOXINS

When Barbara's father was diagnosed with Alzheimer's disease, she got rid of every aluminum pot, pan, and serving container in her parents' home as well as her own. "I read that accumulations of aluminum have been found in the brains of people who had Alzheimer's, so I'm wondering how much of a role it played in my father's case?"

Barbara's question is a good one. We know that concentrations of aluminum in serum increase with age, but it's uncertain whether the aluminum accumulates slowly over time or is more easily absorbed as people age. Higher serum levels of aluminum have been found in some people who have Alzheimer's disease compared with people who have other types of dementia or who are dementia-free.

At this time, however, no study has definitively linked aluminum with Alzheimer's disease, and I find the results of studies that try to implicate aluminum in Alzheimer's disease to be unconvincing. If switching from aluminum cookware to another material makes you feel safer, there's no harm in doing so.

THE BOTTOM LINE

Among scientists and medical professionals, it's generally agreed that a combination of genetics and various lifestyle and environmental factors are involved in the development of Alzheimer's disease. The best thing anyone can do is to accept the risk factors that can't be changed, and modify those that can.

We offer many suggestions on preventive measures in chapter 5, "A Pound of Prevention." But first, we turn to a discussion of the methods I and others use to diagnose Alzheimer's disease.

Chapter 4

Uncovering Alzheimer's Disease

Many doctors still consider a diagnosis of Alzheimer's disease to be one of exclusion—that means they rule out everything else that could be causing the signs and symptoms and then they diagnose Alzheimer's disease when they've run out of options. I believe, however, that more and more Alzheimer's disease is a diagnosis of inclusion. Although it's true that there is no single, comprehensive clinical test that can definitely diagnose Alzheimer's disease, it's also true that **we doctors currently have at our disposal many effective tests and tools that, when used appropriately, allow us to identify Alzheimer's disease with up to 95 percent accuracy.** In fact, even five years ago in a research study that colleagues and I published in the *Archives of Neurology,* we were able to predict Alzheimer's disease with an accuracy of 84 percent.

The key words here are "when used appropriately." In assembling the clues that may or may not lead to a diagnosis of Alzheimer's disease, physicians often function like detectives solving a mystery. We use all the appropriate tests and tools to gather all the relevant clues and then weigh the information carefully so we can accurately "solve the mystery." Relying too heavily on one or two clues can lead physicians astray. For example, I have several patients whom I diagnosed as having Alzheimer's disease, and they have had that diagnosis for five years or more, yet they can still easily pass many of the standard cognitive tests physicians often use to help diagnose the disease. If I had relied heavily on the results of those tests early in the diagnostic process, these individuals would not have received an accurate diagnosis and, as a consequence, they would not have received early intervention with treatments that have allowed them to continue to function so well.

In this chapter I discuss the various diagnostic techniques that you may encounter when you visit your physician or a memory disorder clinic to uncover the reason behind persistent memory problems. These techniques typically include taking a thorough medical, medication, and family history, a physical examination, neurological testing, various laboratory tests, imaging procedures, a battery of tests to determine level of cognitive functioning, and, in special cases, an electroencephalogram.

Where do you go to begin this process? That's a good question, so in this chapter we explain what to look for when choosing medical professionals and/or a memory disorder facility.

But before even one test can be administered, you must first acknowledge that you or a loved one has a problem that needs evaluation. Because this critical step is often the hardest one people have to take, we begin this chapter with a discussion of that initial acknowledgment and how important it is to you or to a loved one who may have Alzheimer's disease, and then help you find a professional who can help you with your journey.

STEP ONE: ACKNOWLEDGING THE NEED FOR HELP

One thing that prevents people from talking to their doctor about memory problems is fear: fear that the diagnosis may be Alzheimer's disease. Fear is the reason many of my patients and their families initially find it difficult to take the first step and seek a consultation and evaluation. I respect and understand their feelings.

But living with uncertainty and denial can take a huge toll on people's lives. More importantly, it can prevent them from seeking the knowledge that can help them live their lives to the fullest. My message to anyone who is struggling with whether to see a doctor about a memory problem—whether for themselves or a loved one—is this: **Taking that first step is possibly the bravest, kindest, and most empowering thing you will ever do. Being willing to know and accept the truth, to take control of your life (or help a loved one do so), and to say "I care enough about myself and my family to rid ourselves of this fear of uncertainty" is a courageous step.**

If the diagnosis is not Alzheimer's disease—perhaps it's age-related memory loss, mild cognitive impairment, or some treatable cause of memory loss—they can release their stress and work with their doctor to take whatever action is required.

If the diagnosis is Alzheimer's disease, then they can take comfort in knowing that they have identified the problem and can now take immediate steps to slow the progression of the disease and make the lives of their loved ones as full and productive as possible. I find that once individuals take that brave, critical step past denial and fear in search of answers, they feel better because then they at least have some control over the situation. Delay, denial, and ignorance are the worst ways people can deal with the possibility of Alzheimer's disease; action, acceptance, and knowledge are the best.

Remember, delaying treatment for even a few months can

have a significant impact on cognitive functioning. An early diagnosis also gives individuals time to participate in any medical, legal, and financial decisions concerning themselves or their loved ones. This may include deciding whether they want to participate in a clinical study of an Alzheimer's drug, choosing where or with whom they will live, changing a will, or making business decisions.

At the end of this chapter, we will talk more about the positive, hopeful, and goal-oriented approach I take with individuals and their families when the diagnosis is Alzheimer's disease. But for now, let's help you find professionals to work with you.

STEP TWO: FINDING A DOCTOR

Once you are convinced that you need to seek medical help, the question is, to whom do you turn? In many cases, people make an appointment with their primary care doctor or internist, and in today's world of managed health care, this is usually the obligatory first step. Then, in many cases, the physician takes a medical and family history; orders an MRI scan (magnetic resonance imaging; explained below) to rule out brain tumors or stroke; administers a short cognitive functioning test called a Mini-Mental State Exam (MMSE; also explained below); and then decides whether the patient needs treatment. If this approach sounds too simplistic, you're right, and here's why.

This approach, although done with good intentions, dramatically shortchanges both patients and their families. One reason is that these individuals have not received the type of truly comprehensive evaluation that memory problems require.

Another reason is that if the diagnosis is Alzheimer's disease, they deserve a much more aggressive evaluation and treatment plan. **It is my experience that Alzheimer's disease is a condition like diabetes or stroke: it is chronic, it can be treated, and if people make lifestyle changes and informed medication choices, they can live relatively productive, happy lives.** I tell them that I see many patients in my practice who have Alzheimer's disease and who still work, volunteer, care for their grandchildren, travel, and lead active lives.

Yet when patients and their families don't get the comprehensive workup and evaluation they should have, they leave their doctors' offices feeling hopeless, frightened, and alone. Some may have been told they have a fatal disease, that there is no cure, that there are medications that can provide some temporary help, and that eventually they will likely be confined to a wheelchair or bed and need around-the-clock care.

Finally, with this type of evaluation, many of the early cases of Alzheimer's disease would be missed. That's because most physicians rely on the MMSE, a test that is not sensitive enough for most of the cases I deal with. (I explain why under "Mental Status Testing.")

You Deserve a Memory Disorder Specialist

To be fair, not all primary care doctors use this approach we just described, yet many of them do not refer their patients to a specialist. **You have a right to see a memory disorder specialist**, and it is in your best interest to ask for a referral, to either a neurologist, psychiatrist, or geriatrician who specializes in memory disorders; or to a memory disorder facility, which is typically staffed by physicians as well as therapists and social workers, and where you can get the type of aggressive medical treatment and cognitive therapy that I've found to be very effective in people who have Alzheimer's disease. (There's more about my treatment approach later in this chapter, under "Diagnosis Alzheimer's: Now What Happens?")

Shopping for a Specialist

In today's health insurance environment, individuals are often told they must choose their doctors and medical facilities from a limited list. Regardless of the limitations placed on you, it is best to fully explore all your options and learn all you can about the doctors you are considering for your loved one's care. The following guidelines can help you make your selection.

- When you meet with the doctor, does he/she make you feel comfortable? Are your questions answered in a clear and patient manner? Does he/she project a caring attitude? You are possibly going to be establishing a long-term relationship with this person over one of the most stressful periods of your life. Comfort is of utmost importance.
- Time is equally important for a thorough memory evaluation. Do you and your family get to spend enough time with the doctor for this to occur? (Generally about 45 minutes.)
- Does the doctor's office perform, or are they able to refer you for, a good battery of cognitive evaluations? Is the person who performs this evaluation competent and are your results going to be reviewed by your doctor?
- Does the doctor's office staff make you feel welcome? Are they helpful and friendly? We feel the office staff are almost as important to your care as the doctor, passing on messages and ensuring availability in cases of emergency.
- Ask your own doctor and others who they would go to if they had a memory problem that concerned them. This will often get you started on the right track.
- How many years has the doctor been practicing? Specifically, how long has he/she been a memory disorder spe-

cialist? Did the doctor receive any fellowship or subspecialty training in memory disorders?

- Is the doctor board certified? Doctors must satisfy high standards to acquire board certification. Ideally you want a doctor who is board certified in psychiatry, neurology, or geriatrics and specializes in memory disorders. The American Board of Medical Specialties Certified Doctor Verification Service can tell you if a doctor has been certified in a particular field. The service is free and can be accessed at www.abms.org.

STEP THREE: IN SEARCH OF A DIAGNOSIS

You've arrived at the doctor's office, and it's time for the diagnostic process to begin. Not all doctors or clinics will conduct all the tests we discuss below, nor will they necessarily do them in the order we talk about them. We hope you will use this information to better prepare for the diagnostic process so it will be as stress-free as possible for you. To further that cause, we've included several "Take Action" sections in this chapter so you can be more proactive in the search for a diagnosis.

Medical, Medication, and Family History

An accurate diagnosis depends immeasurably on the ability of the patient and the patient's family to provide complete, comprehensive information about the affected individual's medical, medication, and family history. In situations where both patient and family are present, the doctor should conduct three separate interviews: one with the patient alone, one with family members alone, and one with both patient and family present. This approach allows physicians to get a more objective and comprehensive idea of the situation.

Because a patient may have memory loss, there may be a

tendency to marginalize or patronize him or her. Doctors should always include and address patients in all conversations that involve them, no matter their level of disability. There is nothing more humiliating and dehumanizing than being spoken of as if you were not in the room.

The consultation and office visit can be a stressful experience in and of itself. Given the uncertainty you may feel, it's best to prepare for these questions at home, before you see the doctor. This advance preparation will allow you to provide more accurate information. To help you with this task, you can use the checklist in the box as a guide.

Doctor's Questions for Patients and Family Members

Before your doctor's visit, write down your answers to these questions in a notebook and add thoughts and comments as they come to you. Every tidbit of information can prove helpful when making a diagnosis.

- What symptoms have you noticed? (For example, difficulty remembering how to do familiar tasks, misplacing objects, having trouble finding the right word when speaking, difficulty recognizing acquaintances.)
- What is your best estimate of when these symptoms first appeared?
- Have these symptoms changed in any way over time, and if so, how?
- Are the symptoms interfering with daily activities? If so, how? Give some examples. For instance: is the person's forgetfulness affecting his/her job performance? Is the

individual leaving items on the stove and forgetting they are there? Have the person's driving skills deteriorated?

- Are there any other current medical conditions?
- Are there any past medical conditions? Include any history of surgical or medical procedures. In women, was there early menopause or a hysterectomy?
- Is there a history of head trauma where there has been significant injury or a loss of consciousness (e.g., automobile accident, sports injury, fall)?
- What medications are currently being taken (prescription and over-the-counter/alternative/vitamins)? If female, is the individual taking, or has she ever taken, hormone replacement therapy?
- Does or did anyone in the family have memory problems? If so, at what age did it start and what was the diagnosis?

TAKE ACTION: Note that there are questions regarding menopause and hormone replacement therapy in the list. I believe these questions are critical to ask of women who are in menopause. However, the majority of doctors typically either do not *ask these questions, or if they do pose them, the information gathered is not viewed as possibly having an impact on a woman's memory problems. I encourage any woman who is in menopause, who is experiencing memory problems, and who is seeking medical attention to work with a physician who appreciates the role hormones may play in memory loss.*

If your medical history (including medication use) is complicated, it may be helpful to write out or type up your history and bring it in on your visit to give to the doctor to place in your records. I often advise patients to place *all* medications and over-the-counter supplements they take in a bag and bring it in to their visit.

Physical Examination

A thorough physical examination is necessary to look for the presence of any heart, respiratory, kidney, liver, or thyroid problems that could be causing Alzheimer-like symptoms. Your doctor should evaluate your blood pressure and nutritional status (e.g., blood levels of vitamin B_{12}, folic acid, and overall levels for deficiencies or signs of malnutrition) and ask about any other physical complaints you have not already mentioned.

Neurological Examination

During a neurological examination, physicians examine the nervous system for signs of conditions that can affect memory and cognitive abilities, such as brain tumors, stroke, Parkinson's disease, multiple sclerosis, and epilepsy. The tests are simple, painless, and quick, and may include the following:

- Higher cognitive function testing: Testing your ability to understand language, translate ideas into action, and so on.
- Cranial nerve testing: Testing nerves that are responsible for sight, smell, taste, hearing, movement and sensation in your face and neck.
- Coordination test: You may be asked, for example, to touch your extended index finger to your nose.
- Muscle strength: Your doctor may ask you to squeeze her fingers or push against resistance.
- Muscle tone: The request may be for you to move your

arms and legs in a particular way to see if your limbs on different sides of the body respond differently.

- Sensory testing: Use of a tuning fork and other tools to evaluate sensation in different parts of the body.
- Reflex test: Your practitioner may tap your elbow, knee, and other joints with a rubber-headed hammer to determine the level of nerve functioning.
- Gait test: As you walk across the room, your doctor will observe your gait for any abnormalities.

Mental Status Testing

The standard test for determining the status of a person's memory, organizational abilities, and language is the Mini-Mental State Exam (MMSE). This is the test that family practitioners and internists use, and although it is a good screening tool, it isn't sensitive enough. Let me explain why.

Of a possible 30 points, individuals can score 10 points if they know where they are and what the date is. They can score another 11 points if they can spell "world" backwards, can repeat what they hear, and can correctly identify two common objects, such as a watch and pencil. Doctors typically regard any score greater than 21 to indicate that the person is operating at an acceptable mental level, yet I have patients who have advanced Alzheimer's disease who can score 28 on the test. Therefore, the results of the MMSE should be viewed in light of all the other findings during the diagnostic process.

TAKE ACTION: If you or a loved one has a memory problem and your internist conducts the MMSE and says the results don't indicate a problem, but the memory problem still seems to be getting worse, you should insist on a referral to a specialist so you can get a more comprehensive evaluation. Consider this: if you went to an internist complaining of chest pains, the doctor would do a few tests, and even if the test results were negative, because you complained of pain, he or she would refer you to a specialist. Yet if you go to an internist with a memory problem and the preliminary test results are normal despite continuing memory loss, the doctor is likely to attribute it to normal aging and do nothing more for you.

Don't allow yourself to be dismissed.

You have the right, indeed an obligation, to insist on a more comprehensive evaluation if you are experiencing memory problems, just as you would if you had chest pain. Yet I know what stops many people: fear that they're going to discover they have Alzheimer's disease. I know that I emphasized the importance of overcoming that fear earlier in this chapter under "Step One: Acknowledging the Need for Help," but it is important enough to repeat here. I want people to understand that getting a diagnosis of Alzheimer's disease—if indeed that is *the diagnosis—is not the end of their world. It can be treated. Depending on the individual and on how aggressive treatment is, some people do well for the rest of their lives without getting progressively worse. But if we don't diagnose the disease in its early stages, we may lose the chance to curb the progress of the disease and keep the quality of life as high as possible.*

Laboratory Testing

The results of blood and urine tests complement those of the neurological and physical examinations. Blood and urine testing helps physicians identify conditions such as anemia, thyroid problems, infections, kidney and liver disorders, hypoglycemia, diabetes, low levels of vitamin B_{12} and folate (folic acid), and levels of any medications, all of which can have an impact on memory and the ability to think clearly.

I also test for methylmalonic acid (high levels of this substance occur in people who have a vitamin B_{12}/folate deficiency) and homocysteine levels when I'm checking vitamin B_{12} and folate levels to uncover latent deficiencies and because of the propensity for this substance to damage brain cells (see "Homocysteine" in chapter 3). In my opinion, identifying homocysteine levels is important, especially among people who have mild cognitive impairment, a condition that places them at an increased risk of developing Alzheimer's disease. Thus, the earlier high homocysteine levels are detected, the faster I can work with a patient to bring them down using diet and supplements (see "Keep Your Eye on Homocysteine" in chapter 5, and "Folic Acid, Vitamin B_{12}, and Riboflavin" in chapter 8), hopefully to reduce their chance of developing Alzheimer's disease.

Brain Imaging

Your doctor may order a brain imaging test to assist in the diagnostic process. Three different approaches are currently used, and each one offers a different level of sensitivity.

Computerized tomography (CT) scan. Although a CT scan uses an X-ray beam to generate images of the internal body, it provides more detailed information than an ordinary X-ray. That's because the CT scanner takes multiple images as it rotates around your body, and then a computer assembles the images into a highly detailed image. Computerized tomography scans can be used to detect blood clots, stroke, tumors, and other brain abnormalities.

Magnetic resonance imaging (MRI). Unlike an X-ray, magnetic resonance imaging uses radio waves and magnetic fields, which produce clear images of brain structure and changes that occur there. An MRI image provides more details than a CT scan, but it is also more expensive.

The MRI is superior to CT scans for imaging brain structure. It is used to rule out brain tumor, brain abscess, stroke, and other causes of brain abnormalities. It can also indicate a decrease in volume in the hippocampus. However, this finding alone is not a definitive sign of Alzheimer's disease, although it can be weighed along with other findings to arrive at a diagnosis.

A new type of MRI, which uses a three-dimensional video technique that can document minute, sequential destruction of areas of the brain, may become part of the diagnostic process someday soon. According to a recent study (*Journal of Neuroscience,* February 2003), researchers used this new approach (called "functional MRI," or fMRI) to document the progression of Alzheimer's disease in patients over a two-year period. fMRI may eventually become useful for early detection, rate of disease progression, measurement of response to treatment, and differentiating Alzheimer's disease from normal aging. It is not yet ready for routine clinical use.

Positron emission tomography (PET). I use PET scanning for those patients where I need further help to make a diagnosis. Anyone who undergoes this costly technique receives an injection of a type of sugar (glucose) that has been altered to transport a weak radioactive material, which gives out signals that are monitored by detection equipment. The sugar is transported to the brain, which requires large amounts of energy to function. Doctors then use the scanner to observe areas of brain activity versus areas that have been damaged and so are less active. Both CT and MRI scans are not able to provide this type of information, as they are structural studies, as opposed to functional ones.

Again, PET use is reserved for certain situations. For example, Michael, a forty-eight-year-old plumber, came to me complaining of memory problems. His evaluation and neuropsychological battery results were essentially normal, but because he had a strong family history of Alzheimer's disease and persistent symptoms, I ordered a PET to see if there was any indication of the classic pattern for the disease: reduced activity in the temporal and parietal regions. His results came back normal, which allowed me to reassure him. I then suggested that he do brain exercises at least three to four times a week (see chapter 6, "Brain Boosters: An Exercise Program for Mental Fitness"), and we worked together to create a program he could do easily at home.

Although PET is not used routinely to diagnose Alzheimer's disease, the findings of researchers at several different universities and research facilities have been very encouraging and may soon change that. At the University of California–Los Angeles, for example, investigators found that when they injected a special material into patients, they were able to detect brain lesions that appeared before the plaques that are believed to destroy neurons. This finding may eventually help physicians detect Alzheimer's disease much earlier than we can now, and possibly prevent or delay its occurrence.

Single photon emission computed tomography (SPECT). This test detects how blood circulates through the brain, and thus can detect areas where a lack of blood has caused brain cell death. Results of a recent study at the University of California–Davis Medical Center indicate that use of a SPECT scan increases the likelihood of getting a correct diagnosis of Alzheimer's disease. The accuracy of that diagnosis, however, depends on the scan being read by a highly experienced professional. I suggest people ask the imaging center how many brain SPECT scans they do per year. You should choose a center that reads at least a hundred brain SPECT scans yearly. You have a right to choose the center that will perform your scan.

Neuropsychological Evaluation

There are many useful neuropsychological tests that can be administered to help make a diagnosis of Alzheimer's disease, but they are merely a part of a much larger toolbox of diagnostic implements (see box, "Cognitive Testing Tools"). One drawback of these cognitive tests is that each one measures a different function or part of the brain, so a negative result on one or two tests can be misleading. One woman, for example, had been told by a friend that if her mother "failed" the Clock Drawing Test, it was a definite sign that her mother had Alzheimer's disease and would quickly deteriorate. It's unfortunate that some people hear—and believe—such inaccurate information.

Yes, the Clock Drawing Test (see box, "Cognitive Testing Tools") is a useful tool. But I have patients with Alzheimer's disease who can't "pass" this test, yet they continue to function very well in many other areas of their lives. One gentleman, a clinical psychologist, has been diagnosed with Alzheimer's for seven years. He continues to see and competently counsel patients, yet he cannot complete the Clock Drawing Test. Another patient, a civil engineer, can draw a beautiful clock, and he continues to construct for his job as well, but he can't remember names and needs to write down almost everything he hears in order to remember it. If a physician were to give these individuals the Clock Drawing Test and make a judgment on their cognitive abilities based on the results, he or she would be off base.

Therefore, you should know that while these neurometric tests can provide more in-depth information for your doctor to use in his/her diagnostic process, they are only one part of the bigger picture. Another consideration with these tests is that they are not sensitive to differences in educational level, language barriers (e.g., people for whom English is a second language), and cultural/ethnic differences. These factors can make a significant difference in how individuals understand and respond to questions, as what may be viewed as a "wrong" response may simply be the result of misinterpretation or misunderstanding by the patient.

Cognitive Testing Tools

Cognitive testing can offer physicians clues about how the brain is functioning, but the results of these tests are not enough for a diagnosis. If your doctor or memory disorder center orders cognitive tests, here are some of the ones you may encounter:

Mini-Mental State Exam (MMSE): Screens cognitive function. This is a 30-point test, and a score of less than 24 indicates early to mild dementia. Detects problems with time and place orientation, abstract thinking, object registration, recall, verbal and written cognition, and constructional abilities.

Wechsler Adult Intelligence Scale III: Evaluates verbal and visual skills by measuring vocabulary, language understanding, level of concentration, ability to arrange pictures to tell a story, and other tasks.

Wechsler Memory Scale III: Evaluates both verbal and nonverbal memory.

Rey-Osterrieth Complex Figure Test: Evaluates the ability to draw a complex figure from memory.

Boston Diagnostic Aphasia Examination: Tests all aspects of language abilities.

7-Minute Screen: Rates the ability to recall a series of pictures immediately and after a short time lapse; also asks individuals to name as many objects as they can in a specific category (e.g., animals, colors) in a given time period.

Clock Drawing Test: Asks participants to draw a clock and hands to reflect a specific time. Patients with early dementia often misplace and/or omit numbers.

Buschke Selective Reminding Test: Measures short-term verbal memory.

Wisconsin Card Sorting Test: Measures the ability to deduce sorting patterns.

Trail Making Test: Times an individual's attempt to draw a line connecting consecutively numbered dots and measures mental flexibility.

DIAGNOSIS ALZHEIMER'S: NOW WHAT HAPPENS?

Every day across America, hundreds of individuals and their families are called into doctors' offices and are told that they or a loved one has Alzheimer's disease. When most people hear those words, they form a picture in their mind as to what they think the future holds: being crippled in a wheelchair, confined to a nursing home, unable to recognize family or friends, unable to care for themselves. These images often leave them gripped by fear, sadness, and a feeling of helplessness.

Yet when I call a patient and his or her family into my office, my message is very positive. I begin by saying that what I'm going to tell them may sound depressing, but that I really don't see it that way. Does this sound like I'm about to discuss Alzheimer's disease? Let me explain.

Explaining the Diagnosis

Alzheimer's disease is an illness that has been very misunderstood. Despite the gloomy images most people conjure up in their minds, this condition is the best studied and best treated, so far, of any of the memory disorders we have. In past years, a diagnosis of Alzheimer's disease was made when the disease had already progressed, usually, to its moderate stage. Today, however, more people are being diagnosed earlier in the course of the illness, which is the time when we can make a significant difference in influencing the disease and its progression. Thus the earlier we identify and treat the illness, the more likely we are to change its course and help individuals live fuller, more productive lives.

One thing that helps people accept the diagnosis of Alzheimer's is when I make an analogy to stroke, diabetes, or another chronic disease. I explain that some people who have a stroke end up crippled in a wheelchair, but most of them recover to some degree and make lifestyle adjustments and then live relatively productive lives. Alzheimer's disease is a chronic condition, and if people are willing to make changes in their lifestyle and take medications, they too can hope to lead a reasonably productive life. That's when I remind them that I have seen patients in my practice who are still traveling, working, volunteering, and socializing with the same or nearly the same vigor as before they got their diagnosis.

Forming a Plan

I believe it's important to present patients and their families with a complete picture of the illness, including the positive and negative factors of their specific case, and a variety of treatment options. This means I encourage them to look realistically at the future and help them plan for it. Gloria's case is a good example.

Gloria is a seventy-five-year-old retired bookkeeper who received the news of her diagnosis in the company of her two children, Dorothy and Brian. Except for mild arthritis and high blood pressure controlled with medication, Gloria is in good health. I explained that the life expectancy for women is approximately eighty-six years, and so we should plan on how to keep her functional and living independently in her own home for the next eight to ten years. My words surprised Gloria and her children, as they do other patients and families, but as I talk about how we can accomplish this goal, they see that it is possible.

First we discuss the factors that are in their favor. For Gloria, this meant that she was living independently without major problems, and she was told to continue her independent lifestyle. She was also in good physical condition, so I encouraged her to maintain a regular exercise program, such as walking daily. Because she was not experiencing any psychiatric symptoms (e.g., delusions, hallucinations, agitation), there was no need to prescribe any psychiatric medications at the time.

On the negative side, she was having trouble finding the right words, so she was advised to begin cognitive therapy (brain exercises; see chapter 6) to help maintain her language skills for as long as possible. I assured her that the cognitive therapy she would be doing would partly focus on this problem.

If there had been evidence that other parts of Gloria's brain were involved—say, with parkinsonian symptoms such as tremors or shuffling, I would have suggested aggressive physical therapy and possibly a medication that would protect the affected parts of the brain (see chapter 10, "When Alzheimer's Isn't the Only Health Concern"). Likewise, patients who are experiencing some psychiatric problems may need medication to keep them under control.

I review all the test and evaluation results with the patient and the family and let them know that the neurological tests will be readministered in a year to see what changes have occurred from the current, baseline results. Families appreciate this tracking of their loved one's condition, as it makes something intangible (memory loss, trouble with speech, difficulty with abstract thought) more concrete and thus makes them feel they have some control over it.

Talking About Sensitive Issues

Many sensitive issues can arise when patients and families have to deal with a diagnosis of Alzheimer's disease, and one of those issues is nursing home placement. This is a topic I address early with individuals, as it usually involves much careful planning and thought. People want to know: do my loved ones need someone to stay at home with them, or do they need to be placed in a nursing facility?

My policy is to speak with the patient and the family separately on this matter, because sometimes family members are uncomfortable asking about placement when their loved one is present. Most families like to have the separate talk, but some will insist that the patient be in the room as well. Regardless of whether the placement talk is done separately or together, I always make it very clear that the ultimate goal is to keep the patient healthy and as independent as possible.

Another issue I always address is securing an eldercare lawyer. Competent legal advice is a must when you are dealing with Alzheimer's disease, and I tell every patient and/or family to seek the advice of such legal counsel immediately. Such a decision can mean a great deal to patients who are still able to participate in decision-making, as it gives them some control over how their financial, medical, and personal affairs will be handled should they ever reach a point where they need help making such decisions. Until they reach that point, they should be allowed to choose how and where they want to live; whether they wish to participate in drug trials (see chapter 7); and the type of medical, complementary, and psychological care they will receive.

Hands-on Therapy

My dual training as a neurologist and psychiatrist allows me to do cognitive rehabilitation with my patients, and it is something I thoroughly enjoy sharing with them. This is a luxury that very few doctors can pursue, however. In the vast majority of cases, patients work with a psychologist, psychiatrist, or speech therapist separately. The types of tasks we do vary from patient to patient, but they typically can involve reading, vocabulary, math, word games, storytelling, and problem-solving skills. Some of the tasks are described in detail in chapter 6, "Brain Boosters: An Exercise Program for Mental Fitness."

THE BOTTOM LINE

Arriving at a diagnosis of Alzheimer's disease requires that doctors use all the appropriate and relevant tools at their disposal, and then evaluate their findings carefully. Despite the lack of a single test that can identify the disease with 100 percent accuracy, we doctors have a very reliable diagnostic tool chest at our fingertips. But the real work begins after the diagnosis is given: that's when patients and their loved ones enter a new phase of life, one geared toward maximizing potential, cherishing their lives and living them to the fullest, and making plans for the future. It's a time when family and friends can renew their commitments to each other and work together to understand and manage Alzheimer's disease.

Before we look at the various treatment and lifestyle options in part II, we turn to a topic on the minds of millions of Americans: how to prevent memory loss and Alzheimer's disease.

Chapter 5

A Pound of Prevention

Some people say that because we can't cure Alzheimer's disease (yet), we don't know exactly what causes it (yet), and we don't have ironclad proven ways to prevent it (yet), there isn't anything we can do except hope we escape its clutches. I couldn't disagree more.

I believe we know enough about Alzheimer's disease—and we are learning more every day—that everyone can take preventive measures that can be easily incorporated into their lives. I impress this idea upon all my patients and their family members, the latter of whom are often frightened, even terrified, that because Mom or Dad or a sibling has been diagnosed with Alzheimer's, the same fate awaits them just around the corner. And in the vast majority of cases, this just isn't true. In fact, some people worry so much about following in the footsteps of a family member with the disease that they develop memory problems that are solely related to their high level of stress—a clear example of mind over matter!

I want to relieve that stress, calm the fears, and give people practical, convenient, even enjoyable ways to help prevent memory loss and the possibility of Alzheimer's disease. The truth is, two-thirds of what determines successful aging is associated with lifestyle and environmental factors; one-third is genetics. This means you have more control over memory loss, aging, and Alzheimer's disease than you may have thought possible.

In this chapter I will tell you how modest changes in diet and nutrition, exercise, sleep, hormone replacement therapy, stress reduction, and intellectual stimulation can help prevent memory loss and Alzheimer's disease, and I will give you detailed guidance to help you along the way. If any of the guidelines seem familiar, that's because most of them are the same preventive measures you can use to prevent cardiovascular (heart attack, peripheral heart disease, angina) and cerebrovascular (stroke, transient ischemic attacks [TIAs]) disease.

BARELY WORKING UP A SWEAT

Aerobic activity improves the ability to think, remember, and concentrate by at least 5 to 10 percent in people who have Alzheimer's disease. Do you want to reduce your risk of developing Alzheimer's disease by as much as 30 percent? According to the results of the large (more than 4,600 men and women age sixty-five and older) Canadian Study of Health and Aging, regular exercise can do just that.

Another study suggests that exercise can reduce the risk of dementia by as much as 40 percent. The walking habits of approximately 6,000 women were evaluated, and researchers found that those who walked more than 200 blocks per week (10 miles) reduced their risk of dementia by 30 to 40 percent compared with sedentary women.

In a five-year study conducted by investigators at the

University of Washington–Seattle. Linda Teri, Ph.D., and her colleagues found that when people with Alzheimer's participated in a home-based exercise program and stuck with it, they stayed in better physical *and* mental shape over time. Compared with patients who did not follow an exercise program, those who did were also less likely to be institutionalized because of behavioral problems.

Getting Ready to Move

With a little forethought and planning, nearly everyone can find time for regular exercise: 30 minutes of aerobic activity (walking, jogging, bicycling, aerobics class, water aerobics, stationary bicycling, treadmill) four to five times a week. It may mean getting up 30 minutes earlier in the morning, taking a brisk walk during lunch hour, or jogging away your stressful day before dinner.

Aerobic activity gives your body a blast of hormones called endorphins, which not only help memory but also improve mood. Because there is a strong correlation between depression and Alzheimer's disease (see chapter 2), such a mood lift is important to achieve and maintain. Recent studies also indicate that exercise causes the formation of new synapses and blood vessels in the brain, a definite advantage against Alzheimer's disease. Yet another benefit of regular aerobic activity appears to be an improvement in the ability to do problem solving.

A less direct but nonetheless still important benefit of exercise is that it helps reduce the risk factors that can lead to Alzheimer's disease, including high blood pressure, obesity, diabetes, and stroke.

Before you begin a regular exercise program, you should talk to your doctor, especially if you have a medical condition that

could require special precautions. Once you have an okay to begin, keep the following guidelines in mind.

Exercise Guidelines

- Include a warm-up and a cool-down period of gentle stretching (at least 15 minutes for each) with each exercise session.
- Choose activities that you enjoy so you'll be more likely to continue your program. If possible, add a little variety: for example, brisk walking two days, an aerobics class another, and stationary bicycling on two days.
- If you're new to exercise, begin slowly and increase gradually. If you start with 10 minutes of aerobics, after one week increase by 5 minutes every other session, then after another week or two add 5 minutes to the other sessions, and so on, until you reach 30 minutes per session.
- Exercise with a friend when possible. Company makes exercise seem more like a social event. Consider joining an aerobic team activity, such as tennis or racquetball, once a week.
- Wear the proper equipment for whatever activity you choose: good walking or running shoes, a helmet if bicycling outside, pads and a helmet if Rollerblading.
- Incorporate more physical activity into your daily lifestyle: take the stairs, walk to the corner store, opt for a brisk walk before lunch.

SLEEP FOR BETTER MEMORY

If you think losing sleep is no big deal, think again: sleep deprivation, which is a significant problem in today's society, can have a big impact on brain function, as well as your heart. Too little sleep impairs your memory and your ability to think clearly, and it raises your cortisol levels—a stress hormone that is associated with memory loss.

If you feel tired all or most of the time and know you suffer with insomnia (difficulty falling or staying asleep), you should seek help from a sleep clinic to identify the cause of your problem and get treatment. Another sleep-related problem that is associated with memory problems is sleep apnea. More than 10 percent of adults have unrecognized sleep apnea (repeated pauses in breathing lasting at least 10 seconds), and this condition can cause depression and memory loss. Again, a sleep clinic can help you identify and correct this condition.

HORMONE REPLACEMENT THERAPY

The role of estrogen therapy or hormone replacement therapy (HRT, estrogen and progesterone combined) in the prevention of Alzheimer's disease in women is the subject of much investigation. My research, and that of my colleagues, shows that a decline in estrogen levels, which occurs with menopause and hysterectomy, is associated with memory loss and difficulties with attention and concentration. Once I prescribe estrogen (soy-based) for women who demonstrate these cognitive problems, their symptoms virtually disappear.

When it comes to the ability of estrogen or HRT to prevent the development of Alzheimer's disease, some studies show that women who have been taking hormones for ten years or longer have at least a 50 percent decreased risk of developing the disease compared with women who don't take hormones. Because menopause typically occurs when women are in their fifties, and Alzheimer's disease tends to manifest in people sixty-five years and older, women who begin hormone replacement therapy at menopause could benefit from its protective effects.

The Women's Health Initiative Trials

Yet many women are confused and frightened by reports from several trials, including the Women's Health Initiative trials, which shed a negative light on estrogen use and memory in women. In these widely publicized studies involving over 4,500 women between the ages of sixty-five and eighty, researchers found that the use of a horse-derived estrogen and synthetic progesterone drug (Prempro) increased the prevalence of dementia of all types, including Alzheimer's, by *twofold.* In other words, over a five-year period, forty women on Prempro and twenty-one on placebo developed dementia. However, the presence of stroke was higher in the estrogen group; and the use of horse-derived estrogen, as well as the use of progesterone, may be associated with these results. Parenthetically, it is interesting that the use of these hormones did not increase the risk for mild cognitive impairment, which it should do, as this condition is believed to be a precursor to Alzheimer's disease.

The findings in these studies seem to say to women, "Don't take estrogen or HRT because it increases your risk of dementia." In fact, the Women's Health Initiative trials also found that estrogen and progesterone increased the risk of breast cancer and venous thrombosis.

Hormones Can Help Memory

So why do I recommend estrogen and HRT to some women? In my opinion, although these studies are the best of their kind to date, certain factors may have contributed to the startling results. First, the researchers used estrogen derived from the urine of pregnant horses, and this is not the same hormone a woman's body produces. Second, the HRT therapy was a combination of horse urine–derived estrogen and a synthetic progesterone. Neither of these artificial hormones is like those the body produces naturally, and they may not have the same beneficial effects as the natural hormones. Third, the women were sixty-five years and older, older than the age when women normally start to take estrogen or HRT for menopause (which is about age fifty). Finally, many of the women in these studies had high blood pressure, diabetes, or high cholesterol, risk factors not only for heart disease and stroke but also for Alzheimer's disease.

Not all women are good candidates for estrogen or HRT, however. Long-term estrogen use causes an increased risk of breast cancer. Adding progesterone to estrogen may slightly increase the risk of breast cancer. I advise all women who are considering estrogen or HRT to make sure they have a complete personal and family medical history in hand when they discuss this possibility with their physician. The doctor should have a thorough knowledge of the benefits and risks of hormone therapy and use natural hormone products (soy-based estrogen and micronized progesterone, *not* progestin). (See chapter 8, "Complementary and Hormone Therapies," for a discussion on why I use natural hormones.)

FLEXING YOUR NEURONS

Think of your brain as a muscle that needs to be exercised every day. Flexing your neurons is believed to be one of the best ways to ward off memory loss and Alzheimer's disease. Although direct evidence to support the adage "use it or lose it" isn't yet available, there is sufficient evidence to suggest that there is a significantly reduced risk of developing Alzheimer's disease among people who routinely engage in mentally stimulating activities, such as reading, playing a musical instrument, doing puzzles, and writing. Such "brain exercises" appear to increase the number and strength of the connections between the neurons. Mindless activities, however, such as watching television or listening to music, do little or nothing to challenge your brain.

In fact, a study reported in the *Proceedings of the National Academy of Science* in 2001 found that watching television was the primary leisure-time activity of nearly every one of the 193 people in the 555-participant study who had developed Alzheimer's disease. In comparison, the participants who engaged in mentally stimulating activities had more than a 50 percent reduction in risk of developing Alzheimer's disease.

I believe flexing your neurons is such an important factor in preventing memory loss and helping to hold on to memory and cognitive functioning for as long as possible that I have dedicated an entire chapter to it (see chapter 6, "Brain Boosters: An Exercise Program for Mental Fitness").

DESTRESS YOUR BRAIN

Reduction of stress helps prevent direct cell death in the hippocampus, an area of the brain responsible for routing memory. When you consider that the hippocampus loses about 6 percent of its cells every ten years after age forty-five, and that stress can increase that percentage, you should make every attempt to be proactive about reducing the stress in your life.

Stress management can take many forms; for some people physical exercise such as running, tennis, or bicycling relieves their tension. For others, meditation, yoga, tai chi, spending time with their pet(s), listening to music, or deep-breathing exercises do the trick. Whatever method(s) you choose, you should make stress reduction a part of your life and consider it a necessary part of your daily routine. You may find that many of the therapies I discuss in chapter 9, "Stimulating the Senses," are excellent ways to reduce stress.

Staying socially connected with people is an essential part

of stress reduction, because it allows you to share your thoughts and concerns as well as form and maintain emotional relationships. Socialization is particularly important for older individuals, who sometimes isolate themselves, especially if they have lost a partner or are not close to their family. Establishing a social and support network with a church, senior citizens club, volunteer organization, support group, neighborhood club, or other group can make a significant difference in how you manage the stress you experience in your life.

FEEDING YOUR BRAIN WELL

Experts have been studying the effects of diet on memory loss and brain health, and so far they've gathered convincing evidence that there are certain food choices and eating habits best for preventing Alzheimer's disease and for promoting optimal brain and memory function, as well as overall health. Generally, a diet that reduces the risk of stroke, heart disease, obesity, cancer, hypertension, and diabetes is also good for the brain. If this sounds like a great deal, you're right—one approach that helps prevent our greatest disease challenges!

Low Fat, Good Fat

Studies show that a low-fat, good-fat diet is good for your brain. But how "low" is low, and what are good fats?

Low fat. Not all experts agree on the exact percentage of fat that should make up a healthy diet, but the range is 20 to 30 percent. The lower end of that range may look very attractive to you if you consider the findings of a Case Western Reserve University study in which investigators found that young and middle-aged adults who consumed a low-fat diet may significantly reduce their risk of developing Alzheimer's disease.

Another good reason to keep fat intake low is that it helps people keep their weight down. Excess body fat with high cholesterol increases the risk for transient ischemic attacks and strokes, which interrupt blood flow in the brain and can cause memory problems and increase risk for Alzheimer's disease. In addition, more than a dozen studies show that high-fat, high-calorie diets correlate highly with Alzheimer's disease prevalence. One of the most recent studies, published in the *Archives of Neurology* in August 2002, found that people who consumed the most calories and fat had twice the risk of developing Alzheimer's disease than individuals who consumed a lower-calorie, lower-fat diet.

Good fats vs. bad fats. Good fats are those that promote brain health and are beneficial for overall health as well. In the "good fat" category are omega-3 fatty acids, a type of polyunsaturated fat that can be found in olive oil, canola oil, flaxseed oil, and fish oil, green leafy vegetables, avocados, and nuts.

Another reason olive oil, canola oil, flaxseed oil, and avocados are considered healthy is that they provide monounsaturated fat to your diet. Monounsaturated fat helps lower LDL cholesterol (the "bad" cholesterol), which is a contributor to heart disease, stroke, diabetes, and high blood pressure.

In the unhealthy fat category are saturated fats and omega-6 fatty acids (a type of polyunsaturated fat), both of which are found in meat and other animal foods (cheese, ice cream, milk), processed foods, fried foods, and margarine; trans fats (hydrogenated or partially hydrogenated oils or shortening), found in margarines and many fried and processed foods; and vegetable oils, including safflower, sunflower, corn, soybean, and peanut oils.

In particular, research shows that people who have

Alzheimer's disease or other types of cognitive impairment often also have low blood levels of docosahexaenoic acid (DHA), one type of omega-3 fatty acid. It is uncertain whether these low levels could be a risk factor for Alzheimer's disease or if they are a sign of the disease. DHA, which helps reduce the risk of heart disease, is found in high concentrations in fatty fish (e.g., salmon, tuna, herring), fish oils, and omega-3 enriched eggs. Although eating fish several times a week can help, taking supplements of DHA, especially for people who don't like fish or who are vegetarians, is a good choice.

Some studies have shown that people who consume a diet high in omega-6 fatty acids experience more problems with memory and cognitive decline than those who eat a healthier diet. While you don't have to completely avoid foods that are high in omega-6 fatty acids in order to have better brain health, I recommend treating them more as a "condiment" than as a main course.

How to use good fats. The healthiest way to include the good fats (olive oil, flaxseed oil, and canola oil) in your diet is unheated. That is, use them to make salad dressings, drizzle them on cooked vegetables or prepared pasta, or stir them into soups, stews, or sauces right before you serve them. If you decide to use these oils for frying, they do produce fewer cell-damaging free radicals than other oils. The healthiest way to fry with the good fats is to stir-fry: place the oil in your skillet and heat it quickly with your vegetables, rice, or other foods, stir them briskly for about two minutes, and then remove the skillet from the heat.

Welcome Antioxidants

One of the buzzwords of the past decade was *antioxidants,* and it's still a good word to remember when talking about maintaining the aging brain and preventing memory loss and Alzheimer's disease. Antioxidants are substances that fight cell-damaging molecules called free radicals, which cause oxidative stress in the body and speed up the aging process, including declining brainpower. Antioxidants can also help fight inflammation, a characteristic of Alzheimer's disease. To help prevent these signs of deterioration, you should include lots of foods rich in antioxidants in your diet.

Although researchers haven't studied all the many antioxidants and their possible impact on memory, brain function, and Alzheimer's disease, a few have gotten some significant attention. Some of the well-researched antioxidants include vitamins C and E, the mineral selenium, lycopene, and catechin. These and other antioxidants are available in a wide variety of foods (see box, "Antioxidant-Rich Foods"), which is the preferred way to get these nutrients. In fact, several recent studies published in the *Journal of the American Medical Association* showed that taking supplements of antioxidants doesn't provide the same level of protection that consuming antioxidant-rich foods does. Most antioxidants are also available in supplements, however, and they can be taken to enhance the benefits of foods that contain antioxidants.

There is some research to support consumption of antioxidants. For example, in one study researchers noted that among people older than sixty-five years, those who regularly took supplements of vitamins C and E were less likely to develop Alzheimer's disease. In other studies, people who took these supplements had fewer problems with memory or cognitive abilities than those who did not take them.

Antioxidant-Rich Foods

Avocados	Mangoes
Beets	Mustard greens
Blackberries	Onions
Blueberries	Oranges
Broccoli	Papayas
Brussels sprouts	Plums
Cabbage	Prunes
Cantaloupe	Raisins
Carrots	Raspberries
Collard greens	Red bell peppers
Corn	Romaine lettuce
Cranberries	Spinach
Dandelion greens	Strawberries
Eggplant	Sweet potatoes
Garlic	Tea (green and black)
Grapefruit	Tomatoes
Green bell peppers	Turnip greens
Kale	Watermelon
Kiwi	Yams

What about selenium? Results of animal studies support the use of this mineral as a way to protect brain cells. Strong evidence of the brain-protective abilities of selenium in humans is not yet available. To test this theory, a large (10,000 older adults) eight-year study of selenium and vitamin E was initiated in late 2001.

The benefits of another antioxidant, catechin, can be enjoyed if you consume tea. Studies of green and black tea have shown that they can help prevent vascular disease such as stroke, and that they have an anti-inflammatory benefit as well. Both of these features make tea (regular or decaffeinated) a healthy choice of beverage. Experts don't agree on the exact number of cups per day that is most beneficial, although many recommend drinking at least three.

If tomatoes are one of your favorite foods, you're in luck. Tomatoes are the best source of an antioxidant called lycopene, which, based on the results of several studies, appears to be especially protective against cognitive decline with age. Topping the list of lycopene-rich foods is tomato paste, followed by spaghetti sauce, tomato sauce, tomato ketchup, tomato soup, tomato juice, vegetable juice, and canned tomatoes. One study found that women who ate only 1 ounce of tomato paste per day for three weeks reduced the damage of free-radical activity by 33 percent. You can increase the benefits of lycopene if you consume these foods with a small amount of healthy fat, such as olive oil or olives. One easy way to combine tomatoes with a healthy fat is in a dish of pasta served with tomato sauce made with tomato paste, olive oil, and black olives.

If you decide to enhance your intake of antioxidants with supplements, you should talk to a professional who is knowledgeable about nutrition before you take them. Generally, for healthy individuals, doctors recommend 400 to 800 IU (International Units) of vitamin E daily, as this antioxidant is more difficult to get from foods. I typically recommend a much higher dose of vitamin E as a treatment for Alzheimer's disease (see chapter 9). For vitamin C, 500 to 1,000 mg daily is typical, depending on your consumption of vitamin C–rich foods. A typical dosage of selenium is 50 to 100 micrograms (mcg). There are no specific guidelines for taking catechin or lycopene.

Keep Your Eye on Homocysteine

You may recall our discussion of homocysteine in chapter 3, where we learned that people who have high levels of homocysteine are twice as likely to develop Alzheimer's disease as those who have low levels. One effective way to keep those levels down was recommended by the researchers involved with the DASH (Dietary Approaches to Stop Hypertension) study: eat foods daily that are rich in folate (folic acid), which include green leafy vegetables, citrus fruits and fruit juices, beans, and whole-wheat breads, cereals, and pastas.

Although folic acid is an essential element in keeping homocysteine at a reasonable level, this nutrient needs a little help from several B vitamins—B_6 and B_{12}. Vitamin B_6 is found in cereals, vegetables, and bananas, while vitamin B_{12} is found primarily in animal products such as fish, meat, and milk, or in cereals and soy products that have been fortified with the vitamin. Because many people older than sixty have a reduced ability to absorb vitamin B_{12} properly from their food, a sublingual (a supplement that is taken by placing it under the tongue and allowing it to dissolve) B_{12} supplement is recommended. Ask your doctor for the best dose for your needs.

Go Light on Sugar

The average American consumes more than 130 pounds of sugar a year, and all that sweetness is not so sweet to the body and the brain. Excess sugar can be converted by the body into saturated fat, which is bad for your brain and your heart. A high-sugar diet can increase free radical activity and damage brain cells, which contributes to memory loss. Sugar also makes your body less able to successfully fight off infections, which makes you more susceptible to bacterial and viral conditions that can reduce quality of life.

How much sugar is too much? According to the U.S. Dietary Guidelines, established by the U.S. Department of Agriculture, the average person should consume no more than the equivalent of 10 teaspoons of sugar per day. Yet most people have no idea how much sugar is in the foods they eat. If you really want to know, you can calculate sugar content by reading the nutritional panels on the package. Look for the sugar level in grams. Four grams of sugar equals 1 teaspoon of sugar. You may be surprised to learn that one 12-ounce can of regular cola contains about 11 teaspoons of sugar; one cup of plain yogurt, up to 5 teaspoons; a tablespoon of jelly, 4 to 6; ½ cup of unsweetened applesauce, 2; and most commercial cupcakes with icing, 5 to 6.

The Alcohol Dilemma

When it comes to alcohol, it appears that while heavy drinking is devastating for brain cells, moderate consumption can be helpful. Several large European studies found that people who drank moderately (one to two drinks daily) had a lower risk for developing memory loss and Alzheimer's disease than people who didn't drink at all, or those who drank heavily. Studies done in the United States (where moderate drinking is defined as two drinks daily for men and one for women) also show that people who drink wine lower their risk for developing these problems.

The alcohol of choice is red wine, which experts believe is helpful because it contains high levels of antioxidants. Beer, in fact, may be associated with an increased risk of developing dementia.

Although red wine appears to be a preventive factor in Alzheimer's disease, if you do not drink, I'm not suggesting that you start. However, if you currently consume alcohol, you may want to adjust your consumption habits, especially if you are drinking heavily.

Caffeine: The Two-Edged Sword

When we think about memory loss and Alzheimer's disease, caffeine is a substance that has both advantages and disadvantages, which means it can be a double-edged sword. On the positive side, the Canadian Study of Health and Aging found that, in addition to regular exercise, regular consumption of coffee also can help reduce the risk of developing Alzheimer's disease. If you are a coffee, tea, and/or caffeinated soft drink consumer, you're probably glad to hear that caffeine can have a positive effect on the brain.

Caffeine provides an energy boost, enhances mood, reduces fatigue, and increases attention. It can also improve the ability to recall, but this is a short-term benefit. It is believed that caffeine stimulates brain cells to make choline, a substance needed to make acetylcholine, a brain chemical that is reduced in people who have dementia. Thus caffeine indirectly raises levels of acetylcholine in the brain.

On the negative side, caffeine can cause insomnia, nervousness, and irritability and may precipitate migraine attacks. Therefore, if you don't consume caffeine now but you start later, you may experience these symptoms. If you drink caffeinated beverages every day and you try to quit, you'll discover that it can cause physiological dependency. Abruptly stopping intake of caffeine can cause headache, migraine, fatigue, depression, and problems with concentration. These symptoms can last for days or weeks. If you are accustomed to getting a caffeine "fix" every day and you even significantly reduce your intake, you may experience some temporary problems with memory or concentration.

The bottom line is, if you are consuming caffeinated beverages and they are not causing you any problems (insomnia, irritability, stomach upset, nervousness, headaches and migraines), there is probably no reason to change your habit unless you want to. If you don't drink caffeine products, there's also no reason to start and risk experiencing possible side effects.

Summary of Dietary Guidelines

To keep the brain—and body—as healthy as possible, I encourage my patients to follow these simple guidelines:

- Avoid, as much as possible, the bad fats (saturated fat, trans fat, omega-6 fatty acids), which are found primarily in meat, poultry, dairy products, mayonnaise, margarines, fried foods, and some commercial salad dressings.
  - If you eat meat, choose the leanest cuts, trim off excess fat, and limit intake to 2 ounces or less daily.
  - If you eat poultry, do not eat the skin, as it is very high in fat. Limit intake to 2 ounces or less daily.
  - If you eat dairy products or mayonnaise, choose no-fat or low-fat varieties
  - If you eat margarine, look for trans fat–free spreads, such as Smart Beat and Smart Balance.
  - Instead of buying commercial salad dressings, you can make your own using olive oil, flaxseed oil, or canola oil. There are some commercial brands that use these healthy oils, such as Newman's Own and Annie's Naturals.
- Use good fats, such as flaxseed oil, olive oil, and canola oil, unheated (see "How to Use Good Fats").
- Reduce intake of animal protein and focus more on plant proteins, which are free of cholesterol and saturated fat.

Some excellent plant protein foods are soy products (tofu, soy milk, miso, textured vegetable protein), beans, quinoa, tempeh, split peas, and lentils.

- Keep sugar intake to a minimum. Try these tips to reduce sugar intake while satisfying your sweet tooth:
  - Avoid foods that are obviously sweetened with sugar (cookies, candy, cakes, soda).
  - Read labels. Many processed foods have high amounts of sugar. (Remember that ingredients are listed in descending order, with those most prevalent listed first.) Breakfast cereals, canned soups, peanut butter, ketchup, salad dressings, yogurt, and fat-free foods (in which sugar is added to make up for the reduced amount of fat) often harbor lots of sugar.
  - Eat fresh fruit instead of reaching for a sugary food.
  - Consider using the herb stevia, a natural sweetener that has virtually no calories. It's available in natural food stores and some mainstream groceries and comes as a liquid and granulated.
- Eat at least five, and preferably seven or more servings of antioxidant-rich fruits and vegetables daily. A serving equals 1 cup raw vegetable, ½ cup cooked vegetable, 1 medium piece of fruit (the size of a tennis ball), or ½ cup cooked fruit.
- Try to get 25 to 30 grams of fiber in your diet daily. Fiber helps slow the rate at which sugar enters the bloodstream, which helps keep blood sugar levels steady. It also helps with weight control, as fiber-rich foods are more filling, and helps keep the intestinal tract in good working order. Foods rich in fiber include whole-grain breads, oatmeal, fresh fruits and vegetables, oat bran, beans, lentils, and split peas.
- If you drink alcohol, red wine appears to provide some benefits. Limit consumption to no more than two drinks

per day (6 ounces per drink) if you are a man and one drink if you are a woman.

NONSTEROIDAL ANTI-INFLAMMATORY DRUGS

Several promising studies have indicated that people who take certain nonsteroidal anti-inflammatory drugs (NSAIDs; e.g., ibuprofen, naproxen, but not aspirin) for at least two years have up to an 80 percent reduced risk of developing Alzheimer's disease. One fifteen-year study, by the National Institutes of Health, found that people who took ibuprofen for as little as two years had half the risk of developing Alzheimer's disease as people who did not take the drug. The study that reported the 80 percent reduced risk was done in the Netherlands and looked at approximately 7,000 people over seven years. Those researchers also found that people who took NSAIDs for one to twenty-three months had an average of a 17 percent reduced risk. I believe a 50 percent reduction in risk with long-term use of NSAIDs (two years or more) is a more accurate figure. Do note, however, that a recent study of NSAIDs for the *treatment* of Alzheimer's proved ineffective.

NSAIDs don't come without health risks, however. Chronic use of these drugs can lead to peptic ulcers and kidney damage. If you are already taking NSAIDs as treatment for a medical condition, you may be reaping the benefits of preventing Alzheimer's disease as well. However, we still do not understand much about the relationship between NSAID use and Alzheimer's disease and so I do not recommend chronic use of these drugs as a preventive measure, nor do I endorse starting to take these drugs solely for the purpose of reducing your risk of Alzheimer's disease. At this point, NSAIDs are continuing to be investigated as a treatment for Alzheimer's disease (see chapter 7 for more details about NSAID use).

THE BOTTOM LINE

If you're worried about losing your memory or developing Alzheimer's disease, your worrying raises your stress level and actually can make your memory worse. Turn your concerns into positive actions like those discussed in this chapter, and you'll get comfort from the fact that you're being proactive in preserving your brain health.

PART II

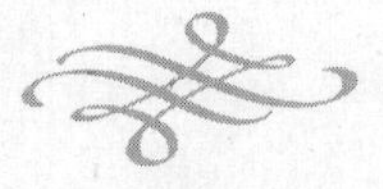

LIVING, REALLY LIVING, WITH ALZHEIMER'S DISEASE

Chapter 6

Brain Boosters: An Exercise Program for Mental Fitness

If you want to keep your heart healthy, you need to exercise regularly. If you want to keep your brain healthy and your memory sharp, you need to make your neurons work hard. This chapter explains how to exercise those neurons—a process I call "brain boosters," or cognitive rehabilitation—both for people who have Alzheimer's disease and for those who want to help prevent memory loss.

I am a firm believer in the adage "use it or lose it" when it comes to memory and cognitive functioning. I also believe, contrary to what many people think, that you are never too old to learn. Brain cells die as a natural part of the aging process, and if the number of brain cells declines, so does the number of synapses between the brain cells. That process can be significantly slowed, however, when brain cells are consistently stimulated and forced to perform, especially those in areas involved with language, motor skills, and memory. When you make your neurons work harder, as you do when you practice a task over and over again, you strengthen the connections (synapses) between the neurons.

In my practice I have many individuals who come into the office once a week for one-on-one cognitive rehabilitation, but here I have designed some exercises for those who would like to be in charge of their own therapy. The brain boosters "homework" is designed to exercise mental muscles in certain areas of the brain (the frontal, temporal, parietal, and occipital lobes we discussed earlier in chapter 1) and help keep cognitive functioning at its best for as long as possible. The tasks are designed to be enjoyable, and I encourage patients to approach them as a game or leisure activity and not "work."

Before we get into a detailed discussion of brain boosters, I want to share Karl's story with you. Karl is a seventy-four-year-old retired banker who was diagnosed with Alzheimer's disease in 1995 by his internist. When he came to see me in 1997, he and his wife of more than fifty years, Emiline, were very distressed. Karl, who had always been an avid reader and who loved to tinker with painting and carpentry, could no longer read or enjoy his crafts. We discussed brain boosters, and Karl and Emiline were willing to give it a try. Karl immediately began an intensive program of what he likes to call "mental gyrations," and slowly but steadily, he improved.

"I was a vegetable before, and now I've learned how to read again, how to write again," said Karl. Emiline is thrilled. "Now he follows TV, music, art, movies; he's aware and interested in what's going on in the world," she said. "We can travel, enjoy theater and interacting." It's been more than six years since Karl walked into my office, and he continues to enjoy life to the fullest.

TYPES OF BRAIN BOOSTER EXERCISES

There are literally thousands of brain booster exercises you can do, but I have chosen twenty-eight as representative samples. The exercises are arranged in a workbook format and categorized according to the type of functioning that needs work: language, working memory, visual/perceptual skills, and life skills. There are more exercises available, including printable and CD versions, at www.nymemory.org.

Language Brain Boosters

Language is housed in two major areas of the brain, with connections between them. The expressive part of language is represented in most people in the left frontal lobe, while the ability to understand is present in the back of the left temporal lobe. Surprisingly to most people, language functions are often involved in conditions like Alzheimer's disease. In fact, I often focus more on maintaining language skills than on maintaining memory skills because I feel they are more important for independent functioning, and that is a major goal of therapy.

Memory Brain Boosters

Memory is stored in many places throughout the brain. The ability to walk and move is stored in regions of the brain called the basal ganglia and cerebellum (see Figure 1 in chapter 1). The ability to recognize faces is stored in the frontal lobes, the ability to remember a poem in parts of the language cortex, the ability to recognize a smell in the temporal lobe, the ability to remember a type of touch in the parietal lobe, the ability to recognize an object in, among other areas, the occipital lobe. The gatehouse for the input, storage, and retrieval of memory is the hippocampus, which, as I mentioned in chapter 1, is the first area to be damaged in Alzheimer's disease. Because memory can be stored in so many places, I focus on the particular types of memory that an individual needs to work on rather than worry about which part of the brain is being worked.

Visual/Perceptual Brain Boosters

The ability to synthesize visual information appropriately is important for daily living. Such information is necessary, for example, to know how to put on your jacket, how to sit in a chair, how to find your way around the block in your neighborhood, and how to tie your shoelaces. Naturally, these and other skills are ones you want to maintain. The ability to perform these skills is based in the parietal and occipital areas of the brain, which work closely with the frontal lobe. Logic and abstract functioning is also housed in this brain region.

Life Skills Brain Boosters

These are more basic skills that involve everyday tasks. Persons who need help with these skills may either have a severe dementia, or, alternatively, be suffering from an apraxia—loss of the ability to do learned movements, despite the desire or physical ability to do so—despite only a mild dementia. Such movements can include grasping a toothbrush, winking, licking the lips, or clapping hands. I want to emphasize that any number of tasks can be taught and reinforced. In one of the most famous cases in medical history, a patient who had had both his temporal lobes removed was taught new tasks, such as playing cards. He got better at it with each session, although he did not recall ever having seen the particular task ever before! Learning was occurring at a preconscious level.

The exercises in this category are usually not done until individuals demonstrate signs that tasks such as eating, getting dressed, bathing, or other daily living activities are becoming confusing. Such difficulties are usually noticed by caregivers and should be mentioned immediately to the doctor so arrangements can be made to begin life skills exercises.

GETTING STARTED WITH BRAIN BOOSTER EXERCISES

As I've worked with patients and brain booster exercises over the years, I've found that **if you set high expectations, patients will rise to them.** This applies also to anyone who doesn't have Alzheimer's disease but who wants to help prevent memory loss.

If you use these exercises to help prevent memory loss, concentrate on those in the first three categories and spend 30 minutes per day, at least three times a week, focusing on language, memory, and visual/perception skills. I suggest that individuals who have Alzheimer's disease spend about 15 minutes three times a week.

If you or a loved one has Alzheimer's disease, ask your doctor to identify the areas in which you need to focus your attention and to suggest exercises in those areas. In some instances, concentrating on shoring up available skills, rather than working with debilitated skills, may be more worthwhile. However, you will certainly benefit by working in all three areas.

Most exercises discussed in this chapter can be done by patients themselves, without assistance from a caregiver, and this is the way I believe they should be done. (Those in the "Life Skills Brain Boosters" are an exception; see above.) People who take charge of their cognitive rehabilitation are more motivated and feel more in control of their lives. In my practice, many people who have Alzheimer's who consistently do their brain booster exercises maintain a high level of functioning for many years.

Getting Help

If individuals need assistance with their therapy, they have two options. One, caregiver(s) can help them. Often, however, caregivers are already stretched to their limits physically, emotionally, and mentally, and adding this task can be overwhelming. In addition, some patients resent being "taught" or helped by their caregiver. Therefore, when I have patients who had been handling their own brain booster exercises but who now need assistance, I generally recommend that caregivers retain a speech therapist, occupational therapist, psychologist, or other rehabilitation professional, depending on the patient's needs. Professionals at a memory disorder clinic (see the Appendix) or stroke or head injury rehabilitation center, which also employ individuals who can conduct this type of therapy, can be of assistance. Ask your doctor or hospital for a recommendation, or contact the Alzheimer's Association for assistance (see the Appendix). Most insurances will reimburse for these types of treatments for at least three months a year, and sometimes longer.

Brain Booster Notebook and Calendar

Some of the exercises require you to write things down, so I suggest you get a spiral-bound or three-hole-punched notebook or binder in which to keep your exercises. Keep similar brain booster exercises together in their own section (e.g., all pages containing work on Brain Booster #1 should be in one section separated by a divided page or tab from the other exercises). This will allow you or your loved one and/or doctor to monitor the exercises. Put the date on all exercise pages.

A brain booster calendar can help you keep a record of all the brain booster exercises you or your loved one engage in. This can be any calendar—a wall, desk, or notebook type—with space adequate to record the type of activities completed on any given day. You may choose to note the activities by number; say, Brain Booster #1 and #15 on Monday; #3 and #20 on Wednesday; and #8 and #18 on Saturday. Or, you may simply identify the type completed: 1 Language and 1 Visual on Monday; 1 Language and 1 Memory on Wednesday.

Instructions

Each brain booster exercise has its own specific instructions. Overall, however:

- Pick activities that you find enjoyable.
- Choose a different activity at each session during the week. Varying the exercises not only helps maintain motivation and keeps interest high, but also works the neurons a little harder.
- If you have suggestions for other exercises, discuss them with your physician before adding them to your routine.
- Have fun!

LANGUAGE BRAIN BOOSTERS

The ability to communicate effectively is, in my opinion, even more important than maintaining strong memory skills for independent functioning. The exercises in this section focus on strengthening both written and verbal communication skills. Despite the fact that they seem like games, these brain booster exercises are really working the neurons hard.

Brain Booster #1: Syllables

Equipment Needed: Notebook, pencil or pen, watch, clock, or timer

Suggested Frequency: Once a week

What to Do: In your notebook, draw a line down the center of a page. On the top of the left-hand side write "Four-Syllable Words," and on the right-hand side write "Five-Syllable Words." Think of as many four- or five-syllable words as you can and write them down in the appropriate column. Allow yourself a set amount of time, say, 15 minutes, and time yourself with a watch or clock. Add up the total number of words in each column at the end of the allotted time.

Tips: Try these ideas to jump-start your brain:

- Look around the room you are in: are there any objects that are four or five syllables long? Is there, for example, a refrigerator (five syllables) or a television (four syllables)?
- Think of specific categories. For example, think of fruits: one four-syllable fruit is watermelon. How about wild animals? A hippopotamus and orangutan each fit into your lists.
- Think of places you traveled to or places you would like to visit. Have you ever been to California? Saskatchewan? Here are two more for your lists.

Things to Consider: Each time you do this exercise, see if you can write down more words than you did the prior session. Do not refer back to the previous sessions' work when you are creating your new list. See if you are repeating some of the same words in each list and/or if you are adding new words at each session.

Brain Booster #2: Anagrams

Equipment Needed: Notebook, pencil or pen, watch, clock, or timer

Suggested Frequency: Twice a week

What to Do: In your notebook, write a polysyllabic word, like "paraphernalia," at the top of a page. Then write down as many words as you can make from this word when you move the letters around. Try to make words that are at least three letters long. You can use proper names (names of people, places, things) as well as foreign words. For example, "hernia," "nail," "pear," and "air" are words that can be made from "paraphernalia" when you rearrange the letters. See how many words you can write in, say, 15 minutes.

Tips: Here are some polysyllabic words, as well as a few words made from them to get you started, that you can use at different sessions. Feel free to add some of your own; you can look in a dictionary or take words from something you are reading. This is an exercise you may want to come back to several times a day.

Administration: station, mini, ration, mind
Anthropocentric: cent, poet, acorn, raccoon
Autobiographical: auto, graph, photo, tool
Bacteriological: logical, bacteria, glacier, broil
Depolarization: polar, deport, ratio, trapezoid
Epidemiological: logical, mold, gloom, damp
Individualistic: dual, individual, vial, last
Participatory: party, tapioca, captor, tray
Rationalization: ration, nation, lion, riot
Sentimentality: sentiment, mental, timely, listen
Totalitarianism: total, talisman, militant, raisin

Things to Consider: The goal is to write down as many words as you can. This exercise really challenges the brain, so if you start to get tired or discouraged, put the exercise aside after you've worked on it for more than 15 minutes and try again later in the day.

Brain Booster #3: Categories

Equipment Needed: Notebook, pen or pencil, watch, clock, or timer

Suggested Frequency: Once a week

What to Do: In your notebook, write the name of a specific category at the top of the page; for example, "Wild Animals." For 15 minutes, write down as many items as you can in that category.

Tips: When you begin to write down words in the category you've chosen, you may get "stuck" after a while. Say you've chosen "Wild Animals" and you've listed twelve animals but can't think of any others. You could stimulate your mind by asking yourself the following questions. Some of the questions may not apply if you have not visited the places mentioned.

- What types of animals have I seen at the zoo?
- What types of animals have I seen at a circus?
- Which animals live in Africa?
- Which animals have I ever seen in the wild in my state? While on vacation?
- Which animals do some people hunt?

Another way to jump-start your brain is to take each letter of the alphabet and think about which animals begin with that letter. For "A," for example, you might say "aardvark," "anteater," and "antelope." For "B," you might list "bear," "buffalo," and "baboon."

Here are some categories you can use for your sessions. Feel free to add others. Automobiles, birds, flowers, trees, countries, dog breeds, vegetables, women's names, men's names, fish, mammals, sports teams, colors.

Things to Consider: Make each list as exhaustive as possible in the time allotted.

Brain Booster #4: Word Associations

Equipment Needed: Notebook, pencil or pen

Suggested Frequency: Once a week

What to Do: In your notebook, make a list of five to ten nouns, one word to a line, down the left side of the paper. Leave several blank lines between each word. Then list five words that are associated with each of the nouns.

For example, if one of the nouns you chose is "Polar Bear," you might list the following associated words: white, furry, Alaska, North Pole, mammal.

Tips: If you need help making a list of nouns, here are some ways to get ideas:

- Look around you: what's in the room or space you're in? Perhaps a couch, lamp, bookshelves, stereo, or recliner? If you're outside, you may see an automobile, elm tree, mailbox, garden, or ranch house. Here are ten words to get you started!
- Picture in your mind your favorite place to visit: what do you see? Perhaps you enjoy the beach: nouns you could list might include sand dunes, seagulls, conch shells, umbrellas, and waves.

- List five or ten gifts you would like to receive or give to someone else.
- List five foods in your refrigerator or pantry and five items in your bedroom closet.
- List five nouns that begin with "A" and five that begin with "B." You can continue at each session using two different letters of the alphabet for up to thirteen weeks!
- List five things you'd find in a grocery store and five things you'd find in a hardware store.

Things to Consider: Write down five words that are associated with each of the nouns. You may choose to begin with just five nouns rather than ten. Then, at subsequent sessions, add one noun each time until you reach ten nouns. If you find it easy to list five associated words for each noun, challenge yourself and try to list ten or fifteen.

Brain Booster #5: Essay

Equipment Needed: Notebook or separate essay book, pencil or pen, watch, clock, or timer

Suggested Frequency: Once a week

What to Do: In your notebook or essay book, choose a topic that interests you and write an essay about it. Spend at least 30 minutes putting down your thoughts on paper. You may want to spend a few minutes jotting down some basic thoughts or a rough outline before you begin your essay. Then let your thoughts flow.

Tips: Stuck for an idea? There are probably dozens of topics that interest you, but how do you pick one? You can pick a topic that is very narrowly focused, such as "Why I Enjoy Raising Violets," or one that is broader, such as "Why I Enjoy Flowers." You may want to comment on situations concerning politics in the United States or abroad, your feelings on space travel, football, classical music, or air pollution. Perhaps you'd like to write about your grandchildren, your favorite pet, why you love chocolate, or your favorite movie of all time. Still stuck for ideas? Try beginning your essay with one of the following phrases:

If I were president, the first thing I would do is ______
If I could travel anywhere in the world, I'd go to ______ because ______
The best day I ever spent in my life was ______
The secret to a good marriage is ______
My fondest childhood memory is ______
The most important thing in life is ______

Things to Consider: Spend at least 30 minutes with this exercise. Your goal is to stay as focused as you can on the topic and put down as many relevant thoughts as you can in a narrative form.

Brain Booster #6: Daily Reading

Equipment Needed: Items to read that interest you, be they romance novels, mysteries, biographies, financial reports, books on gardening, or the newspaper

Suggested Frequency: Daily

What to Do: Spend at least 30 minutes per day reading. If possible, do your reading in one session, but if you find that difficult, you can split it up into two 15-minute sessions per day.

Tips: Everyone has a different attention span and ability to maintain focus when reading, so choose an environment that is best for you.

- Make sure you have sufficient light.
- Don't be distracted. In order to concentrate, some people need complete silence when they read; others feel more comfortable when there is some background music or a low level of activity. Select the environment that works best for you.
- Choose a comfortable position. Do you have a favorite recliner, chair, couch, or lawn chair you like to use for reading? Don't read lying down, however, as it's too easy to fall asleep.

You may want to make reading aloud part of your reading sessions. Francine, a sixty-seven-year-old grandmother of two, spends 30 minutes reading aloud to her grandchildren twice a week.

Things to Consider: Thirty minutes of reading every day is a challenge for some people; for others it's less than they normally do. If you fall into the former category, your goal will be to reach 30 minutes per day. You may start with a smaller goal; say, if you begin at 15 minutes three days a week, gradually work up to 30 minutes three days a week over a month or two, then set another goal of 30 minutes five days per week. Once you achieve that, set another goal of 30 minutes per day. If you fall into the latter category and 30 minutes per day is not a challenge for you, you may decide to read for 60 minutes per day, or simply continue your normal reading habits and choose another brain booster exercise in this section.

Brain Booster #7: Crossword Puzzles

Equipment Needed: Crossword puzzles, pencil, crossword dictionary (optional)

Suggested Frequency: Once or twice a week

What to Do: If you are new to crosswords, begin with less challenging ones and gradually increase in level of difficulty until you feel challenged but not frustrated. (Hint: The *New York Times* crosswords are *not* beginner caliber.) I suggest you do crosswords in pencil, so you can always erase an incorrect entry. Using a crossword dictionary can be helpful, and looking up words is an exercise in itself.

Tips: Crosswords can be found in several different media: puzzle magazines and books can be purchased from bookstores, many department stores, and through the mail. Most newspapers also have a daily crossword puzzle. If you have access to the Internet, there are crossword puzzles available online as well.

Things to Consider: Spend 30 minutes per session working on crosswords, using a dictionary if needed. The goal is to complete the crossword you have chosen. Some crosswords come with target finishing times. Do not feel discouraged if you do not finish the crossword in the time stated.

Brain Booster #8: Word Scrambles

Equipment Needed: Word scramble puzzles, pencil, notebook

Suggested Frequency: Once or twice a week

What to Do: Word scramble puzzles (e.g., "songreain" can be unscrambled to form the word "reasoning") can be found in daily newspapers as well as in puzzle magazines and books. Those in magazines and books may be grouped according to level of difficulty. If you are new to word scramble puzzles, choose those at the easier levels and, if they are not challenging, move on to more difficult ones. Beginner word scrambles typically consist of four or five letters to unscramble. When doing word scrambles, at first try to do each puzzle mentally, without writing down the letter combinations. If this proves too difficult, then work the word out on paper. Begin by working on five to six scrambles per session, and gradually increase to fifteen or twenty.

Tips: To help you solve word scrambles, look for certain clues. For example:

- The combination "ed" is a common ending, and if these two letters appear in the scramble, you might begin by looking for a word that ends in "ed."
- Look for consonants that often appear together, such as "st," "ch," "br," "th," "ght," "pr," and "tr."
- Some vowels commonly appear together, such as "oa," "ai," "ea," "ee," and "ou."
- Common endings include "ing," "ly," and "tion."
- If there are word scrambles you are having difficulty solving, put them aside and go back to them later in the session or even later in the day. Sometimes when you come back to a difficult scramble later, the word "pops" out at you and is obvious.

Here are a few words for you to try. The answers are listed below.

1. eylla
2. nabir
3. nepoh
4. csufo
5. gleba
6. ccouh
7. ldieat
8. rnrtue

Things to Consider: See how many word scrambles you can

solve in 30 minutes. You may begin with five or six scrambles that contain four or five letters and then gradually work up to fifteen or twenty scrambles that contain more letters.

Answers: 1. alley; 2. brain; 3. phone; 4. focus; 5. bagel; 6. couch; 7. detail; 8. return

Brain Booster #9: Describe It

Equipment Needed: none

Suggested Frequency: Once a week

What to Do: Pretend you have a guest who is visiting from a foreign country. This individual has never seen or heard of certain objects that are common in your life. In great detail, describe each object aloud. You might include the following information:

- What the object is
- What it is used for
- Who would use it
- How the object is made
- How it works
- What it smells/tastes/feels/sounds like
- The history of the object

Tips: Examples of objects you can talk about include ice cream, toothbrush, refrigerator, clock, teddy bear, light bulb, microwave, automobile, computer, bagels, toaster, wheelbarrow, telephone, apple, shoes, couch. If you are having trouble getting started, pretend you are talking to a child who has never seen or heard of the object before now. You could pretend to be a teacher who is introducing a new object to a class, or a tour guide who is explaining the object that is in a museum exhibit.

Things to Consider: The idea behind this brain booster exercise is to practice putting into verbal language, in a focused and structured way, the ideas that are in your head.

MEMORY BRAIN BOOSTERS

As I mentioned earlier, memory is stored throughout the brain, so the following brain boosters are designed to tap into those many places. Unlike language skills brain boosters, which can be fun and invigorating, memory exercises can often be frustrating for individuals to do. That's because you are essentially both student and teacher at the same time. For example, if you were to listen to a five-minute speech, wait a few minutes, and then write down the main points of the talk, there's no way for you to know if you got it "right" unless someone else checked what you wrote. However, the mere act of drawing upon your short-term memory and writing down what you recall works the neurons in the brain. Therefore I strongly encourage people to do memory brain boosters.

Brain Booster #10: Poetry

Equipment Needed: Short poetry, eight to twelve lines

Suggested Frequency: Two to three times a week

What to Do: Choose a poem that means something special to you and try to memorize it. Begin with a short poem, perhaps eight to sixteen lines. If you've never tried to memorize poetry before, see the tips below for help. If you choose a sixteen-line poem, you may want to begin by working on the first eight lines only. Because repetition is critical when trying to memorize something, you should practice your poem at least two or three times a week for about 15 to 20 minutes per session.

Here are three short poems to get you started:

Fire and Ice
By Robert Frost

Some say the world will end in fire,
Some say in ice.
From what I've tasted of desire
I hold with those who favor fire.
But if it had to perish twice,
I think I know enough of hate
To say that for destruction ice
Is also great
And would suffice.

I Wandered Lonely As a Cloud
By William Wordsworth

I wandered lonely as a cloud
That floats on high o'er vales and hills,
When all at once I saw a crowd,
A host, of golden daffodils;
Beside the lake, beneath the trees,
Fluttering and dancing in the breeze.

Continuous as the stars that shine
And twinkle on the milky way.
They stretched in never-ending line
Along the margin of a bay:
Ten thousand saw I at a glance,
Tossing their heads in sprightly dance.

The Walrus and the Carpenter (a portion only)
By Lewis Carroll

"The time has come," the Walrus said,
"To talk of many things:

Of shoes—and ships—and sealing-wax—
Of cabbages—and kings—
And why the sea is boiling hot—
And whether pigs have wings."

"But wait a bit," the Oysters cried,
"Before we have our chat;
For some of us are out of breath,
And all of us are fat!"
"No hurry!" said the Carpenter.
They thanked him much for that.

"A loaf of bread," the Walrus said,
"Is what we chiefly need:
Pepper and vinegar besides
Are very good indeed—
Now, if you're ready, Oysters dear,
We can begin to feed."

Tips: Look for poems that rhyme or that evoke pleasing images in your mind. Perhaps there are some poems you remember reading in high school or college that bring back fond memories.

People memorize things in different ways. You might try to memorize the first line alone before tackling the second one; or you may find it easier to recall them together, especially if they rhyme. Some people like to visualize the words in their mind and can memorize poetry in this way. Others prefer to repeatedly write down the lines they wish to memorize, as the act of writing them down helps make the words "stick." Still others set the words to a melody. Choose any approach that works best for you.

Things to Consider: To memorize a poem that you can recite comfortably without referring back to the written copy.

Brain Booster #11: Novel Review

Equipment Needed: At first, a short novel; later, a notebook and a pencil or pen

Suggested Frequency: Varies; depends on how long it takes for you to read a novel. One short novel a month is a good goal.

What to Do: Select a short novel and read it. Choose one that has at least three or four characters. After you have finished the book, write down the major events and characters' names and any distinguishing characteristics about them in your notebook. Wait a day, turn to a new page in your notebook, and make your list again. Do not refer back to the first list. Wait a week, turn to a new page in your notebook again, and make your list again. Remember, don't look back at the lists you've already made!

Tips: Here are a few tips to make this brain booster exercise more enjoyable!

- Choose novels that are fun to read.
- Choose novels that don't have a lot of characters: more than six or eight main characters is too confusing.
- While you're reading the novel, don't keep telling yourself, "I've got to remember this or that," because the stress of trying so hard may make you forget. Read to enjoy.
- Read some of the novel each day (see Brain Booster #6), and quit before you get too tired. If you allow yourself to get tired, you're more likely to forget what you've read.
- You might combine this brain booster exercise with Brain Booster #6.

Things to Consider: Try to read one short novel per month. After you make your lists for each book, look back to see how much you remembered about the characters and events. Do not get upset if you remember less in your second or third list for each book than you did for the first list. Choose a new book and try again!

Brain Booster #12: Autobiography

Equipment Needed: A notebook separate from the one you've been using for your other brain booster exercises; pen or pencil

Suggested Frequency: Two or three times a week, for about 30 minutes each

What to Do: Write your autobiography and include as many details and names as you can. Include addresses, years you moved, names of neighbors and friends, jobs held, memories of special vacations, family gatherings, and so on. This can be an ongoing project, one that you work on several days a week.

Tips: Writing an autobiography is a big project, and there will likely be many memories you'll want to get down on paper. To help you organize the project, here are a few hints:

- Make a general outline of what you want to include in your autobiography. An outline can be very helpful in organizing your thoughts. You might ask yourself:
  - Where do I want to begin: with my childhood? Teen years? Marriage?
  - Do I want to include information about my parents' childhoods and years up to my birth?
  - What information do I want to include about my siblings?
  - What are the most interesting events in my childhood? Teen years? College years? During my twenties, thirties, and so on?

    - What were the two most important events in my life and what happened?
    - Who influenced me most in my life and how?
    - What have my dreams in life been, and which ones have I achieved and how? Which ones didn't I achieve and why?
- Look in old photo albums, yearbooks, and other memorabilia that may help trigger some memories and ideas for your autobiography.
- Talk to family members and friends about the past and ask them for memories of you in your younger years and for their perspective on past events.

Things to Consider: This brain booster exercise involves organizing, writing, and planning, and while it works the neurons hard it is also a labor of love. Some people find this project so satisfying that they have it typed and put into a notebook for other family members to read as well. Others have included photographs. This is an exercise that is highly personal and rewarding for patients.

Brain Booster #13: News Reporting

Equipment Needed: Notebook, pencil or pen, radio or television

Suggested Frequency: Two to three times a week

What to Do: Listen to a short radio or television news broadcast lasting about five minutes. Wait a few minutes and then write down the main points of the broadcast and anything else you can recall.

Tips: While listening to the broadcast, shut out any distractions. Concentrate solely on the broadcast and pay attention to any key words or phrases that are especially poignant or memorable. These may help you recall other points about the broadcast when it comes time for you to write down the main features.

Things to Consider: Write down as much as you can remember about the broadcast. With practice, you may find it increasingly easier to focus in on key words or phrases that will help you better recall the content of the broadcasts you listen to.

Brain Booster #14: Geography

Equipment Needed: Blank map of the United States or Europe without the names of countries and cities printed on them; pencil or pen. Such maps can be purchased at map stores or some bookstores or educational supply shops.

Suggested Frequency: Once a month

What to Do: If you get a map of the United States, write in all the names of the states and, if you know them, the capital of each state. Do not worry about placing the capital in the correct spot within each state—just naming the capital is sufficient. If you get a map of Europe, do the same for the countries and their capitals.

Tips: It's probably been a long time since most people have opened up a geography book, so this exercise can be more challenging than many people think. If you are having difficulty naming the states, try to remember a time when you might have traveled from state to state and the route you took. This may help you fill in some of the states' names. You might also think about things you can associate with certain states. For example, states that border Canada have very cold winters. Which states are traditionally snowbound in the winter months? Similarly, which states are known to be hot and sunny much of the year? You might also divide the map into three or four sections and focus on one portion of the country at a time, as the exercise will seem less overwhelming that way.

Things to Consider: To correctly identify as many states/countries and their capitals as possible within 20 to 30 minutes.

Brain Booster #15: Window-Shopping

Equipment Needed: Notebook, pencil or pen. You will need to leave the house for this exercise.

Suggested Frequency: Once a week or every two weeks

What to Do: Choose a commercial location where you can walk safely—perhaps with a friend—such as a shopping mall or along a commercial street in your town. As you walk, take mental notes of the buildings, stores, and other attractions. Do this for about 15 to 20 minutes. When you get home, make a list of all the sites you saw during the 15 to 20 minutes. Wait a week or two and return to the same mall or street and repeat the exercise.

Tips: There are tricks you can use to help yourself remember the sites along the way:

- Group the sites you see into categories. For example, you may walk past clothing stores (e.g., Annie's Closet, The Gap), restaurants (e.g., The Bistro, Charlie's Café), churches (e.g., St. Mark's Presbyterian, Holy Angels), and office buildings (e.g., Ford Building, Greene Office Plaza). When you say the category name to yourself, this may trigger the names of the sites in that category.
- Create word associations with the sites. For example, on the first block you may see Annie's Closet, The Gap, and the Greene Office Plaza. You can create a short sentence to help you remember the names, such as, "There was a

green gap in Annie's closet." Don't be afraid to be silly; silly often helps you remember!

- Set the names of the sites to the melody of a familiar song.
- Don't worry about remembering. If you are under stress, you are more apt to forget. This should be a fun outing.

Things to Consider: The goal is to challenge yourself to remember as many sites as you can and to find ways you can help yourself remember them. We've given you a few tips, but feel free to create your own.

Brain Booster #16: Movie Review

Equipment Needed: Notebook, pencil or pen; a movie—on television, a rental, or at the movie theater

Suggested Frequency: Once a week

What to Do: Choose a movie, preferably one you have not seen before, and watch it. When it is over, write down the plot, the names of the characters, and the characters' physical characteristics.

Tips: Relax and enjoy the movie. If you try too hard to remember something about a particular character or scene, you may miss part of the story.

Things to Consider: Challenge yourself to remember as much about the plot and characters as you can. Don't worry about getting it "right"; if you have difficulty remembering some of the plot or character traits, do the best you can and try another movie next week.

Brain Booster #17: Math Works

Equipment Needed: Notebook, pencil or pen. You will need to visit a grocery store for this exercise.

Suggested Frequency: Once a week

What to Do: This is a brain booster exercise you can do while grocery shopping. While in the store, mentally add up the cost of the items you put into your cart. Set a goal; say, you'll add up the cost of five items before you write down the total. Increase the number of items you add mentally each time you shop. Although this is a math task, it also stimulates working memory.

Tips: Start with low-priced items (less than one dollar) if possible; for example, $.89 plus $.59 equals $1.48. There are two ways you can approach this exercise. One, you can add up each item as you place it in your basket. If you choose this approach, you can repeat the first total to yourself several times, as needed, until you select the next item you will add to the total, and so on, until you have added up five items. Two, you can do all your shopping, then choose five items from the basket whose prices you will add up mentally.

Things to Consider: To be able to mentally add up the correct total for at least five items in your shopping cart. Once you can add up five items successfully in two or three trips, increase the number you add up mentally to six, then seven.

Brain Booster #18: Grocery Shopping

Equipment Needed: Notebook, pencil or pen. You will need to visit a grocery store for this exercise.

Suggested Frequency: Once a week

What to Do: When you go grocery shopping, choose one aisle and concentrate on the brand names and types of products in that aisle. When you get home, write down in your notebook the different products you can recall. The next time you visit the same supermarket, concentrate on that aisle again and make another list when you get home.

Tips: Focus on the theme(s) in the items in the aisle you have chosen; for example, are there vegetables, pastas, or cereals? Do the products come in cans, boxes, jars, or all three? When you look at brand names, can you associate them with commercials you've seen or jingles you've heard advertising the products? Have you tried any of the items?

Things to Consider: Try to remember as many products as you can in each aisle. You can compare your first list for, say, Aisle 1, with your second list and see what you may have remembered in the second list that you did not in the first, and vice versa. As you return to the store and try this exercise with other aisles, try different tips you may have learned from doing this exercise to help you remember more items.

VISUAL/PERCEPTUAL BRAIN BOOSTERS

The brain boosters in this category are probably the ones that involve the most artistic creativity, although you certainly don't have to be an artist to do or enjoy them. Some patients say that these exercises can't be "homework," because they're too much fun!

Brain Booster #19: House Design

Equipment Needed: Drawing paper (any large [11 x 17 inch is usually adequate] plain paper will do); pencil, ruler, colored pencils if desired

Suggested Frequency: Once or twice a month

What to Do: Draw the floor plan of the place you or a family member live in. Put in all the rooms as well as the furniture, appliances, windows, doors, and so on. If applicable, also include any outdoor landscaping, such as shrubs, flower beds, gardens, and trees. You may choose to color in some of the items on the plans. At subsequent sessions, you may choose to draw the floor plans for places you've lived in the past; perhaps your childhood home, your first apartment or house, or other locations you moved to throughout your life. You can also draw the plan for any other home with which you are familiar, such as that of a close friend or neighbor.

Tips: You don't need to be a draftsman or architect to do this exercise. Just have fun with it.

- Once you have drawn the main outline of the place you live in now, begin filling in the rooms one at a time. You may decide to do one room a day, and so stretch this brain booster exercise out over a week or two.
- You can be as detailed as you wish to be; for example, you may draw a circle to indicate a table that sits next to the sofa, or you may go one step further and draw legs on the table. If there is a lamp on the table, you may place an "X" in the circle to indicate it.
- If you decide to draw the plan for a house you lived in in the past, approach the plan in the same way you did for the house you're in now: one room at a time. Now, however, it may help to sit quietly with your eyes closed and visualize each room as vividly as possible before you begin to draw.

Things to Consider: Do the best you can recreating the floor plans for your current residence or those in your past. Some patients find that doing this brain booster exercise brings back some memories that help them with other brain boosters, such as writing an essay (Brain Booster #5) or writing their autobiography (Brain Booster #12).

Brain Booster #20: Origami

Equipment Needed: Pieces of color paper, cut into squares, 6 x 6 inch or similar size. Origami paper is available at most craft stores. It is usually colored on one side only, but you can also use paper that is colored on both sides.

Suggested Frequency: Once a week

What to Do: Origami is a Japanese art in which paper is folded to resemble objects such as birds, flowers, geometric shapes, toys, and animals, among other items. The best way to learn origami is to follow the step-by-step instructions in books on the subject, or to have someone demonstrate it for you. Several books to get you started include:

Easy Origami, by John Montroll
Bringing Origami to Life, by John Montroll
Complete Origami: An A–Z of Facts and Folds, with Step-by-Step Instructions for over 100 Projects, by Eric Kenneway

These books can be purchased in bookstores or borrowed from the library.

Tips: If you have never done origami before, it is easier to use origami paper, which allows you to distinguish between the two sides of the paper when making your folds.

Things to Consider: You can create some wonderful objects with origami. Some patients make decorations for Christmas trees or gift boxes; others keep a collection of their different creations. Origami is popular around the world, and there are even origami museums and shows that feature these unique pieces of art.

Brain Booster #21: Jigsaw Puzzles

Equipment Needed: Jigsaw puzzle (choose one with a number of pieces that is not overwhelming; 500 is the average number); table on which to assemble the puzzle; good lighting

Suggested Frequency: At least once a week; better daily

What to Do: Choose a table for assembling the puzzle that is big enough for the completed puzzle, plus allows room to spread out the pieces. The location you choose should also have good lighting, either from a lamp or overhead. Work on putting together the puzzle for at least 20 to 30 minutes per day. Many of my patients find that they enjoy going back to work on the puzzle several times throughout the day. This is an excellent way to keep the neurons working.

Tips: If you have never assembled a jigsaw puzzle before, start with a moderately difficult one, say, 500 pieces, and choose a scene that is pleasing and not too complex. A scene that has too many bright colors or that is very intricate can cause eyestrain and be confusing. Begin by assembling the border and then choose a corner or side from which to begin filling in the puzzle with the other pieces.

Things to Consider: Many people are surprised at how relaxing working on a jigsaw puzzle can be. Some say it gives them a sense of accomplishment and order; others say they enjoy watching the process of something being created before their eyes.

Brain Booster #22: Still Life

Equipment Needed: Drawing paper; pencil, charcoal, or pastels

Suggested Frequency: Once a week

What to Do: Draw simple objects such as a book, table, hat, spoon, clock, or cup within a specified amount of time, say, 5 minutes. Choose one or two different items to draw each week. Keep a copy of your drawings in your notebook and date each one. After a few weeks, go back and redraw objects you drew previously.

Tips: Don't worry about drawing something "perfectly"; this is merely an exercise designed to work your ability to translate what you see onto paper.

Things to Consider: You could include some of the objects you draw here in Brain Booster #19, but on a smaller scale.

Brain Booster #23: Tangrams

Equipment Needed: A tangram is a geometric puzzle consisting of between seven and twelve or more geometric shapes (see Figure 3). You can purchase a tangram at a hobby store or at school supply stores, which sell geometric-shaped puzzles based on the same concept as tangrams.

Suggested Frequency: At least once a week

What to Do: The object of a tangram is to arrange the pieces in various ways to create shapes. The pieces must touch but they cannot overlap. There are literally thousands of ways to re-arrange these shapes to look like any type of object—a bird, car, dragon, house, snowflake, or anything imaginable. You can let your imagination go wild.

Tips: If you've never worked with tangrams before, it is helpful to look at shapes other people have created. The book *Tan-*

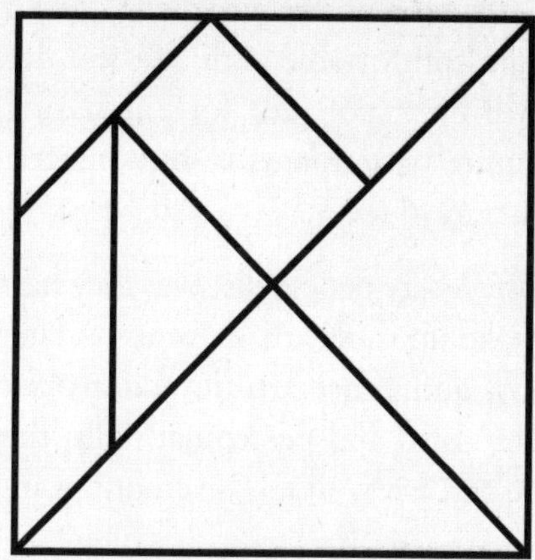

Figure 3: A tangram

grams: The Magnificent Seven Piece Puzzle, by Barbara Ford, has many illustrations.

Things to Consider: When you work with tangrams, you are participating in an ancient art form. There are tangram enthusiasts around the world who practice this art form and who have formed clubs for the purpose of sharing their creations.

Brain Booster #24: Take a Class

Equipment Needed: Depends on the class you choose to take

Suggested Frequency: At least once a week

What to Do: Take a class that allows you to explore your creative, artistic side: photography, watercolors, sculpture, pottery, woodworking, beading, quilting. Many communities offer classes at neighborhood centers, schools, senior centers, and private studios. Better yet, sign up with a friend, so you can share your experiences with someone else.

Tips: Before you sign up for a class, get all the details, such as location, times per week, cost, number of people per class, level of difficulty, experience of the instructor, and refund policy. Make sure you are comfortable with all these details. Ask what materials you will be responsible for purchasing for the class; many classes require participants to buy materials in addition to paying a registration fee.

Things to Consider: Many people discover they have "hidden" talents when they take up these artistic ventures later in life. Painting, photography, and other artistic endeavors offer not only ways to stimulate visual and perceptual skills, they also provide hours of pleasure and a way to release emotions in a creative way.

Brain Booster #25: It's Logical

Equipment Needed: Notebook, pencil or pen

Suggested Frequency: Once a week

What to Do: Think of various commonplace activities such as driving or planning a vacation. Break down each activity into its smallest components and place them in logical order. Write the list in your notebook. For example, if you wanted to list the steps for backing your car (an automatic) out of the driveway, the list might look like this:

1. Get into the car.
2. Insert the key into the ignition and turn it away from you (toward the dashboard).
3. Look over your shoulder and in the mirror to make sure it is safe to back up.
4. Put your right foot on the brake.
5. Put the car into reverse.
6. Put your right foot gently on the accelerator.
7. Back up slowly.

Lists for some activities may be much longer. If you make a logical list for planning a vacation to Paris, for example, there will be many items to consider. I suggest you begin with more common activities and then gradually try more challenging ones. Here are a few activities for which you can make logical lists:

- Brushing your teeth
- Making chocolate chip cookies
- Changing a tire
- Making a bed
- Making a grilled cheese sandwich
- Writing a check to the electric company
- Making a restaurant reservation
- Making popcorn

Tips: Many of the things we do in life we do out of habit, without thinking about them. This brain booster exercise forces you to think about each step involved in performing everyday tasks. To help you better focus on the steps needed to complete a chosen task, try these tips:

- Close your eyes and visualize the activity in your mind. Write down each step as you see it in your mind's eye before moving on to the next step.
- Once you have the list written down, review it carefully, step by step.
- Pretend you are giving the list to someone who has never done this activity before. Did you leave a step out?

Let's look at the example of backing the car out of the driveway. It's important to include the fact that you should turn the key away from you. Someone who has never started a car before would probably not know which way to turn the key.

Things to Consider: Complete one logical list at each session.

You may want to have a friend or family member look at your lists to see if they can follow the instructions.

LIFE SKILLS BRAIN BOOSTERS

Life skills brain boosters are a shared experience between a caregiver, therapist, or other helpful individual, and the person with Alzheimer's disease. If possible, the patient should do two or three exercises each day. Practicing these brain booster exercises can be frustrating for both the person who has Alzheimer's disease and the helper. Therefore, it helps to approach these exercises with calm, patience, and a good sense of humor.

Brain Booster #26: Following Commands

Equipment Needed: None

Suggested Frequency: Daily

What to Do: Ask your loved one to follow a series of simple commands. For example:

- Close your eyes and then lift your left hand.
- Make a fist and then smile.
- Take four steps forward and then clap your hands.
- Sit in a chair with both of your feet on the floor and then lift your left foot.
- Sit down and then clap your hands twice.
- Lift both arms up over your head and then stomp your right foot.

Tips: Choose three to five commands to practice at each session. Each command should be done a few times. You can add other commands to the list, depending on your loved one's abilities.

Things to Consider: Do not look at what your loved one does as being right or wrong. If an individual takes only three steps forward instead of four and has trouble clapping, that's okay; let him or her try again. If the person with Alzheimer's disease begins to get irritated or anxious, stop the exercises for a few minutes and resume them when he or she is calmer.

Brain Booster #27: Gestures

Equipment Needed: None

Suggested Frequency: Every day or every other day

What to Do: Ask your loved one to make gestures that depict different activities. For example, ask the individual to pretend to be:

- Sleeping
- Sick with a stomachache
- Rowing a boat
- Brushing their teeth
- Buttering a piece of toast
- Pouring a glass of water from a pitcher
- Writing a letter
- Washing dishes
- Blowing up a balloon
- Bouncing a ball

Tips: Feel free to add other gestures to the list. Choose three to five gestures to do during each session.

Things to Consider: Do not look at what your loved one does as being right or wrong. If an individual has difficulty doing what you've asked, demonstrate the gesture and then let him or her mimic you. If the person with Alzheimer's disease begins to get irritated or anxious, stop the exercises for a few minutes and resume them when he or she is calmer.

Brain Booster #28: Dress Rehearsal

Equipment Needed: Items of clothing: pants, jacket, shirt, shoes, socks

Suggested Frequency: Once or twice a day

What to Do: Have your loved one practice putting on and taking off clothing, such as a shirt, jacket, shoes, and pants. Choose items that match his or her abilities. For example, if your loved one cannot tie shoelaces, use slip-on shoes or ones with Velcro straps. If buttons are too difficult to handle, practice with shirts that have snaps or that go on over the head.

Tips: These exercises can be incorporated into the person's daily routine, but also practice at least one additional time during the day as well.

Things to Consider: If your loved one has difficulty doing what you've asked, offer some assistance, but allow him or her to do as much as possible alone. If the person with Alzheimer's disease begins to get irritated or anxious, stop the exercises for a few minutes and resume them when he or she is calmer.

THE BOTTOM LINE

I find that most people who have Alzheimer's disease who consistently and conscientiously do brain boosters maintain a high level of functioning for many years and at the same time enjoy a better quality of life. Brain boosters have several other advantages as well—they can be entertaining, educational, and just plain fun, not only for individuals who have Alzheimer's disease, but for anyone who wants to keep their neurons in good working order.

Chapter 7

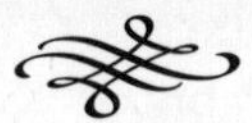

A Pharmacological Approach

How can we treat the brain so memory and cognitive function don't gradually disappear? That is the question scientists continue to ask as they research, test, and develop potential new drugs. Although these drugs are not a cure, when used judiciously and in combination with each other and with complementary approaches, they can be quite effective.

Many doctors prescribe one medication to treat Alzheimer's disease, but I believe this complex disease requires a more aggressive and comprehensive approach, a "two-fisted" approach, if you will. In one hand, the one we will talk about in this chapter, are the drugs that can help us manage both the cognitive and behavioral symptoms characteristic of the disease. I believe that in most cases, one drug isn't enough. In the other hand are the complementary approaches, which I discuss in chapters 8 and 9.

A patient may need one drug to increase the level of acetylcholine (a key brain chemical), another one to protect the neurons from dying, and a third medication that will improve neuronal health. Each patient has his or her own level of functioning and unique needs, so the medication treatment program must be tailored to his or her circumstances and reviewed on a regular basis, preferably at least every two months or when there are behavior or health changes that warrant reevaluation.

Carmela is a good example of how I approach drug treatment with my patients. Carmela is a sixty-five-year-old former ballroom dance instructor who was diagnosed with Alzheimer's disease in 1995 by another physician. At the time, she was experiencing some language difficulties. When she came to see me in 1997, she had been taking tacrine (Cognex) for two years. I continued to prescribe tacrine because she was doing well, but I added vitamin E and estrogen to address her language problems. She improved, but after a year she got very confused, so I stopped the tacrine and switched to donepezil (Aricept). She did well for about a year, but then she became depressed and was experiencing sleeping difficulties. I prescribed paroxetine (Paxil), and her sleep and depression improved. Several months later, however, she became agitated and wouldn't let people help her care for herself, so I stopped the paroxetine and prescribed olanzapine (Zyprexa) for the agitation. The agitation improved, but she was having more difficulties with language and some activities, such as dressing, so I added memantine (Namenda) to her treatment in 2000. She continued to do well on the combination of Aricept and memantine, but then in 2001, she developed a gait impairment, which grew progressively worse over six months. An MRI revealed some accumulated fluid in the brain, a condition called normal pressure hydrocephalus. Carmela underwent surgery to have a shunt implanted into her brain, which drained the excess fluid. Her walking improved almost immediately, and today she plays tennis several times a week.

In this chapter we discuss the currently prescribed drug treatments for the cognitive (e.g., memory, perception, attention, judgment) and behavioral (e.g., apathy, depression, sleep difficulties, psychosis) symptoms of Alzheimer's disease, what results to expect when taking these drugs, and the side effects they can cause. We also consider the role of anti-inflammatory drugs in the treatment of Alzheimer's disease.

HOW TO TREAT COGNITIVE SYMPTOMS

Currently, there are several classes of drugs on the market that can be used to impact the cognitive symptoms of Alzheimer's disease. (Nondrug treatments of cognitive symptoms are discussed in chapter 8.) Let's look at each one separately.

Cholinesterase Inhibitors

Perhaps the most prescribed category of drugs for Alzheimer's disease is the cholinesterase inhibitors. This group includes four medications (trade names Aricept, Cognex, Exelon, and Reminyl) that specifically focus on raising brain levels of acetylcholine, a neurotransmitter that is deficient in people who have this disease. These drugs slow progression of Alzheimer's. In terms of side effects, they all tend to cause similar ones, including nausea, vomiting, diarrhea, stomach pain, and loss of appetite, except for Cognex, which also can cause liver toxicity.

The cholinesterase inhibitors available thus far (there are more under development) are approved by the FDA as only effective for people who have mild to moderate disease. However, they may show promise for those who are in the earliest and later stages of the disease, and they could be of benefit in mild cognitive impairment as well. One large study evaluated the use of Aricept (donepezil) in the treatment of mild cognitive impairment and found that it significantly reduced conversion to Alzheimer's disease.

While cholinesterase inhibitors are not believed to be helpful in persons with severe Alzheimer's disease, in my practice I have maintained patients on them indefinitely because of rapid deterioration in some patients who had stopped taking the drugs. There is now evidence from studies to suggest that stopping cholinesterase inhibitors will result in a decline of function to the level that the patient would have been at if he or she had not been taking the drug. Drugs in this class appear to have an added benefit in improving behavior as well as cognitive abilities.

Donepezil. Donepezil (Aricept) is a drug derived from components of black pepper; it is the most commonly prescribed drug for people who have Alzheimer's disease and the one I prefer in my practice. It works by preventing the breakdown of acetylcholine in the brain. The tablet is taken once daily, which helps with compliance, and it usually causes mild side effects. The typical daily dose is 10 mg, with an increase from a starting dose of 5 mg over six weeks. A common misconception is that the drug works for only about six months, but this is in fact not the case. It continues to work over several years and may have a disease-modifying effect.

This drug is relatively well tolerated, and in more than eight years of practice and with thousands of patients, I've had only about two dozen individuals who had to stop taking the drug because of significant adverse effects, including severe diarrhea and sedation. A common complaint among patients who stay on donepezil is the occurrence of vivid nightmares, drippy nose, and gastrointestinal discomfort caused by gaseous bloating. These problems typically appear once individuals have reached their maximum effective dose and are otherwise tolerating the drug well.

Galantamine. Galantamine (Reminyl) is a drug that is derived from the bulbs of daffodils. It prevents the breakdown of acetylcholine and stimulates nicotinic receptors to release more acetylcholine in the brain. The tablet is usually taken twice a day, and the side effects are similar to those caused by donepezil.

Rivastigmine. Rivastigmine (Exelon) is available in liquid and capsules and is taken twice daily. It prevents the breakdown of acetylcholine and butyrylcholine, a brain chemical that is similar to acetylcholine. The availability of a liquid form is helpful for those with difficulty taking pills. It can then be mixed in with juice or applesauce.

Tacrine. Tacrine (Cognex) was the first drug released to the public for treatment of Alzheimer's disease. In addition to the side effects already mentioned, tacrine can cause liver toxicity, which means people who take this drug must have their blood tested regularly to monitor their liver function. For this reason, and with the introduction of other cholinesterase inhibitors on the market, tacrine is rarely prescribed at this time.

Other Options

Beyond the cholinesterase inhibitors, there are options in a few other drug categories that can be used along with them to complement or enhance the benefits. The decision to use any of these medications is made only after careful evaluation of each individual patient and his or her needs.

Memantine. In October 2003, the Food and Drug Administration approved memantine (Namenda) as a treatment for moderate to severe Alzheimer's disease. This is the first FDA-approved drug for the later course of the disease.

Although memantine was only recently approved for use in

the United States, it has been used successfully for more than ten years in Germany for treatment of dementia. For several years before memantine was approved in the United States, I had been using it in my practice for compassionate and humanitarian reasons, and I have seen some dramatic results.

Kathleen exemplifies those results. I first saw Kathleen in 2000, when she was eighty-four. She had had a history of memory problems for about four years and had experienced several strokes. Her previous doctor had put her on Aricept in 1998, and she was still taking it when she came to see me. I placed her on memantine, along with vitamin B_{12}, folic acid, and a regimen of cognitive therapy. As of early 2003, she was still maintaining an active social calendar and pursuing her love of reading, although she has had some deterioration in her speech.

I captured some visual evidence of the effectiveness of memantine for Kathleen in handwriting samples. Figure 4 shows three samples of Kathleen's handwriting. The top sample illustrates her handwriting before she started taking memantine; it is illegible. The middle sample is an example of her handwriting six weeks after starting treatment; notice the improvement. The last sample is an example of her handwriting one year later; it has remained quite legible.

Before Treatment (9/5/02):

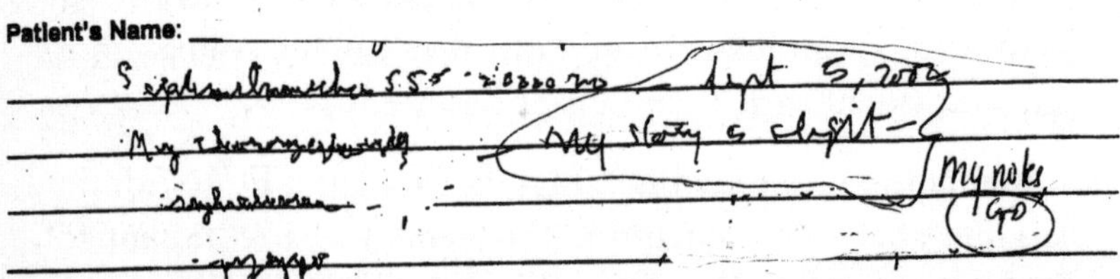

Figure 4: Samples of Kathleen's handwriting before and during treatment with memantine. (*continued next page*)

Six weeks after starting memantine (10/17/02):

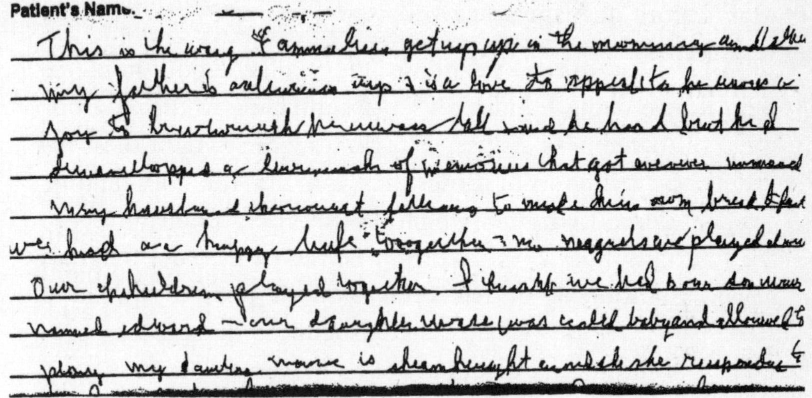

One year later, still on memantine (10/9/03):

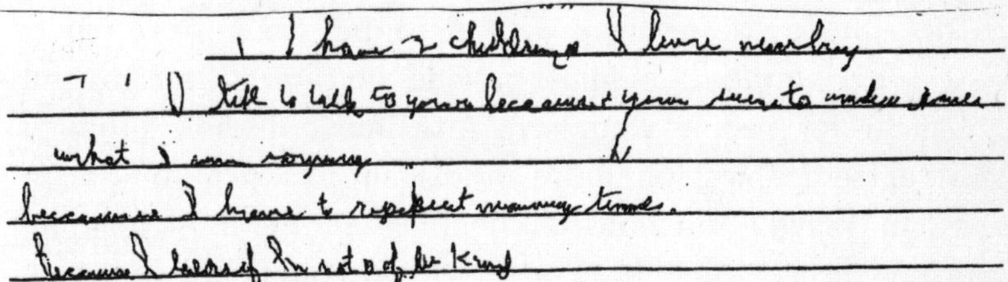

How memantine works. Memantine appears to protect brain neurons against toxicity due to high levels of glutamate, a chemical that is released in large amounts by cells that have been damaged by Alzheimer's disease. Glutamate acts like a key: when it attaches to N-methyl-D-aspartate (NMDA) receptors on cells, it lets calcium enter the cell, which can cause cell damage. Memantine seems to help prevent this damage by blocking the NMDA-docking receptor for glutamate.

Thus far, memantine has been helpful for people who have moderate Alzheimer's disease, and it is my belief that it may be effective in the early stages as well. It can improve cognitive as well as psychological, social, and motor impairments and is generally well tolerated. A 2004 study by Pierre Tariot and colleagues found that memantine enhances the beneficial effects of donepezil in Alzheimer's.

MAO-B inhibitors: selegiline. We've talked about how free radicals can damage brain cells and contribute to the development of Alzheimer's disease, so it makes sense to fight these invaders. Selegiline is a drug that inhibits the monoamine oxidase (MAO) enzyme (which destroys neurotransmitters in the brain) and has antioxidant properties (it destroys free radicals). Traditionally it has been used in people who have Parkinson's disease (which, like Alzheimer's disease, is a progressive neurological disorder), but its potential usefulness in dementia has come to light.

Reports on the effectiveness of selegiline in the treatment of Alzheimer's disease are mixed. According to a 2002 report (*Cochrane Review*), selegiline provides no clinically meaningful benefit for people who have Alzheimer's disease, although other studies have found this antioxidant-like agent to be helpful in delaying functional decline. Perhaps the most convincing evidence came from a large two-year study in which selegiline was found to delay progression of Alzheimer's disease by seven months.

Although selegiline is effective, I prefer to use the antioxidant vitamin E (see chapter 8, "Complementary and Hormone Therapies"), which has excellent free radical–fighting abilities, costs less than selegiline, has similar benefits to selegiline, and has fewer serious adverse effects. However, in patients with parkinsonian features, or other factors related to motor dysfunction, I choose selegiline or another drug in this class. Side effects associated with selegiline include insomnia, confusion, and psychosis.

Nonsteroidal anti-inflammatory drugs. When nonsteroidal anti-inflammatory drugs (NSAIDs; e.g., ibuprofen, naproxen) are discussed, most people associate them with treatment for arthritis, menstrual symptoms, and other health conditions that involve inflammation and pain. Yet NSAIDs appear to play a significant role in the prevention of Alzheimer's disease (see chapter 5), and possibly in treatment, but more studies need to be completed. For now, NSAIDs are not widely used for people who have Alzheimer's disease.

One promising study on the effectiveness of NSAIDs in Alzheimer's disease was reported in March 2003 in *Neuroscience.* Scientists at the University of California–Los Angeles found that common, over-the-counter NSAIDs may dissolve the amyloid plaques—and maybe even prevent the formation of new ones—that are found in the brains of people who have Alzheimer's disease. And there is more evidence:

- A large study by Cornelia van Duijn and colleagues at the University of Rotterdam in the Netherlands found that the use of NSAIDs in higher doses reduced risk for Alzheimer's disease by nearly 80 percent.
- When researchers from the University of Toronto and the University of Washington–Seattle collected data from nine studies that evaluated the use of NSAIDs in nearly 16,000 people with Alzheimer's disease, they found that the drugs tended to decrease the risk of Alzheimer's disease in people who were fifty-five years or older and that the benefits were greater the longer the drugs were taken. Dose levels varied among the studies.

However, a recent study by the Alzheimer's Disease Cooperative Studies section (*Journal of the American Medical Association,* June 2003) did not find either naproxen (Naprosyn) or rofecoxib (Vioxx) to be helpful in treating Alzheimer's disease.

NSAIDs: my caveat. Although several studies provide encouraging news about NSAIDs for people with Alzheimer's disease, we must not forget that chronic use of these drugs is associated with increased risks of stomach and intestinal bleeding, peptic ulcer disease, and renal and kidney problems, especially among elderly people. Therefore, I prescribe NSAIDs only for individuals who have arthritis, a degenerative joint disease, or another inflammatory condition and for whom other remedies don't provide sufficient relief. The use of NSAIDs with any of the cholinesterase inhibitors (e.g., Aricept) should be approached with caution, as the combination increases the risk of gastrointestinal bleeding. Combining these medications can increase the risk of stomach and intestinal bleeding.

Statins. Statins (e.g., atorvastatin [Lipitor], lovastatin [Mevacor], simvastatin [Zocor]) are cholesterol-lowering drugs that work by blocking an enzyme that causes the liver to produce cholesterol. Statins help keep blood vessels healthy and thus are commonly used to prevent heart disease and stroke. Unlike other cholesterol-lowering drugs, statins appear to have a direct effect on the brain. Specifically, they appear to reduce the production of beta-amyloid proteins, which deposit themselves around brain cells and cause damage or death to the neurons. This makes statins possibly good candidates for either prevention or treatment of Alzheimer's disease.

In fact, one study has suggested that statins reduce risk for Alzheimer's by up to 79 percent. In a study of 2,581 people, experts from the Boston University School of Medicine found a 79 percent reduction in risk of developing Alzheimer's disease among people taking statins. There is also increasing evidence that reducing cholesterol levels may slow progression of the disease.

Statins: my caveat. Until more convincing research is done and the long-term effects of statins have been assessed, I'll continue to prescribe statin drugs for individuals with Alzheimer's disease who also have elevated blood cholesterol levels, but I will not recommend them for those who have the disease and healthy cholesterol levels. Statin use has been associated with liver abnormalities, muscle problems, and nervous system damage.

PSYCHIATRIC DRUGS FOR BEHAVIORAL SYMPTOMS

The most pressing challenge for family and friends of people who have Alzheimer's disease is how to manage and cope with behavioral problems; in particular, depression, anxiety, aggression, wandering, hallucinations, irritability, and delusions, among others. When possible, I suggest that caregivers try using nondrug approaches to dealing with these behavioral symptoms (see chapters 9, 10, and 11). In some cases, when a patient does not respond to nondrug methods, a combination of medication and one or more complementary approaches or coping mechanisms is effective. Finding the right combination that works with your loved one may be a matter of trial and error, but with a little patience, success is often possible.

In this section I discuss some of the typical behavioral problems and the various psychiatric medications I find useful in my practice. It's important to remember that everyone has a unique response to psychiatric medications, and elderly individuals are especially less tolerant of them, which means they often experience more serious side effects.

With these facts in mind, I always explain to caregivers that although they may want to see immediate results when a new medication is started, I start at a low dose and increase dosages gradually and carefully so I can monitor the patient's response and tolerance. It can take two to four weeks before a significant change becomes apparent. This approach may be frustrating for caregivers, but it reduces the chance of serious side effects or other problems associated with medication use.

Why Behavioral Problems Happen

Before we discuss the treatment of behavioral symptoms, it is important to understand why patients have these problems. The depression is fairly easy to understand. Patients begin to experience subtle difficulties with their thinking and memory, even though these problems are almost always not apparent to others. They may feel isolated in this situation, worried about seeking help because of fear of being diagnosed with Alzheimer's, and not talking to others about it because of embarrassment. In this stage, they may choose to withdraw from social engagements and settings where their shortcomings may be revealed to others, for fear of exposure. Anxiety accompanies this as well.

Anxiety is also a feature later in the illness, when it can be debilitating to the patient and heart-wrenching and distressing for the caregiver. Later in the course of Alzheimer's disease, patients may become increasingly anxious, growing frantic if they are not with their caregiver or in a familiar environment at all times. Even when they are at home, they may repeatedly ask to go "home." "Home" in this sense is not a geographic location but a symbolic place where one feels comfortable and at ease with oneself. It is this search for home that I believe leads to wandering, another behavior that is a source of great concern for caregivers.

Aggression is a behavioral problem that is a major reason people with Alzheimer's disease are placed in institutional facilities. This aggression is rarely premeditated or planned. It most often is present when caregivers attempt to care for the patient, for instance to bathe the patient, assist with toileting or eating, or to stop a patient from wandering. Patients may then get angry and react as if they are being attacked, as they are not able to understand the reason behind the need to be bathed, for instance. Patients may also be verbally aggressive and irritable because they may feel they are being constantly corrected and belittled. I advocate nonconfrontational techniques for this, and encourage caregivers to pick their priorities when attempting to care for an aggressive individual (see chapter 11).

When medication becomes necessary, caregivers should be reassured there are options. I turn to that discussion now.

Depression

Early in the course of the disease, the predominant psychiatric problem is depression. In fact, patients will often get misdiagnosed as depressed alone when, in fact, they are depressed due to early Alzheimer's disease. Depression among people who have Alzheimer's disease is very common, yet I believe it is often overlooked and thus undertreated. This is unfortunate, as proper treatment can make a significant difference in the quality of life and behavior of patients. As a corollary, many patients with early Alzheimer's disease have depression related to their reduced cognitive abilities and are treated for depression but not for Alzheimer's, thus they lose out on a valuable opportunity for early treatment.

The drugs I find most effective and safe for treating depression among people who have Alzheimer's disease are sertraline (Zoloft), followed by paroxetine (Paxil), trazodone (Desyrel), and bupropion hydrochloride (Wellbutrin), which work well in elderly individuals. Additionally, in a subgroup of patients who are apathetic and appear physically slow, I have found stimulant medications like methylphenidate (Ritalin) to be particularly effective for both depression and cognition.

The most important concern when using antidepressants for people who have Alzheimer's disease is the side effects they can cause. Drugs that are more likely to cause delirium or confusion should be avoided, as these symptoms can significantly affect the quality of life of the person who has dementia. Other side effects commonly experienced by people who take antidepressants include drowsiness, dry mouth, blurry vision, diarrhea, and nausea.

Another consideration is drug interactions. People who have Alzheimer's disease are often taking other drugs, not only for Alzheimer's but for other medical conditions such as high blood pressure, heart disease, diabetes, or arthritis. Your doctor will need to evaluate for possible drug interactions with any drugs being taken for these ailments.

I find that with careful dosing and monitoring of the person's progress with the antidepressant, most problems can be avoided or greatly minimized. Side effects typically occur within the first two to three weeks of starting an antidepressant, so it takes some time before a doctor can determine whether a specific drug is the best choice.

Among the antidepressants I believe should be used with caution by people who have Alzheimer's disease are those in a class known as tricyclic antidepressants, which includes amitriptyline (Elavil) and nortriptyline (Pamelor). These have a higher potential for causing side effects, especially sedation. However, there is a subgroup of patients with insomnia and chronic pain for whom these drugs are particularly effective.

Anxiety, Agitation, and Other Behavioral Disturbances

Perhaps the most disturbing and disruptive behavioral symptoms are those associated with anxiety, aggression, wandering, hallucinations, irritability, and delusions, and therefore these are the ones for which doctors most often prescribe medications known as neuroleptics. Neuroleptic drugs have a sedating effect and help even out a person's behavior, mood, and thoughts.

Agitation was traditionally treated with drugs such as haloperidol (Haldol), which is not as well tolerated in the elderly. Fortunately, newer neuroleptic medications, including olanzapine (Zyprexa) and quetiapine (Seroquel) are now available and have a significantly lower risk for severe side effects. My first choice for people who have agitation as well as insomnia is quetiapine, while olanzapine often helps those who tend to be drowsy or sleepy during the day but who are also agitated. For patients who suffer with severe insomnia as well as psychotic symptoms, I find that a low dose of an antidepressant along with a neuroleptic can be quite effective.

A word about treatment of anxiety. I do not use traditional anti-anxiety medications such as Xanax or Ativan for treating this condition in Alzheimer's patients. I opt instead to use a low dose of an antidepressant or, alternatively, an agent like olanzapine or quetiapine. The anticonvulsant class of medications, including divalproex sodium (Depakote), carbamazepine (Tegretol), and gabapentin (Neurontin) are drugs I also use to control both agitated behavior and anxiety.

The major problem with the use of neuroleptics is development of parkinsonian features, which may predispose patients to falls, fatigue, and sedation. These side effects are especially troublesome in elderly patients.

Apathy

Some experts believe apathy is more common than depression among people who have Alzheimer's disease. Whether or not this is true, apathy *does* affect many patients. Although it can be confused with depression, some telltale indications of apathy are listlessness and a lack of interest, enthusiasm, motivation, and emotion, whereas depressed individuals tend to cry or be tearful, sad, and hopeless.

I find that apathetic patients generally respond well to the psychostimulants methylphenidate (Ritalin) and dextroamphetamine (Adderall).

Sleep Disturbances

People with Alzheimer's disease often experience problems with their sleep-wake cycles. When nondrug approaches aren't effective, I will prescribe a sleeping aid, such as the antidepressant trazodone (Desyrel), doxepin (Sinequan), or the antipsychotic drugs quetiapine (Seroquel) or olanzapine (Zyprexa), as agitation often accompanies sleep disturbances. I stay away from drugs such as temazepam (Restoril), zolpidem (Ambien), and diazepam (Valium) because of their possible interference with memory function and because, paradoxically, in some individuals they can cause agitation.

How to Take Medications

The single most common problem I encounter among patients with early Alzheimer's disease who live alone is ensuring that their medications are taken correctly. Oftentimes, it is for this reason alone that families are obligated to hire a home companion, which may anger the patient, as it unintentionally humiliates him or her by affronting their sense of dignity.

The traditional Sunday-through-Saturday medication dispensers may be difficult to open and may be dropped, which results in the medications becoming mixed up. One method I have used with good success is the following:

- At the beginning of the month, the patient, caregiver, or we at the office gather together all the patient's medications, prescription and alternative, and place each day's supply in a sealed small envelope (obtained at local stationers).
- The date of each day of the month, the day of the week, and the time the medication is to be taken are printed on labels and placed on the front of the envelopes. This allows us to closely monitor medications and to assess compliance and response to treatment.
- With patients who are on more than once-a-day regimens (which I go to great lengths to avoid), each envelope for the day contains two or more smaller envelopes, again each with the date and the time to be taken on it. This method works well as long as it is carefully explained to the patient that the purpose of this approach is not to patronize or infantalize, but to promote optimal independent functioning.

PARTICIPATING IN CLINICAL TRIALS

At any given time, there are typically many clinical trials in progress throughout the United States that are exploring treatments for Alzheimer's disease. A clinical trial compares a specific treatment (drug or complementary approach) with a placebo (sugar pill). Participation in a clinical treatment study is an option some patients and their families consider. If you would like to know more about clinical trials, you should express your interest and questions to your physician. Here is some background information about the pros and cons of clinical trials to prepare you for your discussion with your doctor.

Pros

- If the new treatment under study is shown to be effective, and you are taking it, you may be among the first to benefit from it.
- Clinical trials are monitored very closely and participants typically receive high-quality care.
- You have the opportunity to help others and to improve treatment possibilities.
- Participation in a clinical trial allows people to take a more active role in their treatment.
- Typically there is no charge to the patient or family for any of the treatments, examinations, or other related factors associated with the study. In some cases, in fact, there may be some small monetary compensation for travel and time.

Cons

- You may be among the patients who are given the placebo and not the new treatment being tested. Therefore you would not enjoy the benefits of the new approach.
- New treatments may have side effects that researchers do not expect or that may be worse than those caused by the standard treatment.
- There are no guarantees. Depending on which treatment you receive (drug or placebo), you may not be helped by either one.
- Some studies require many visits to a specific facility for testing. This may be difficult for some people to manage and may require a time commitment by a caregiver or other individual.

Safety

Clinical trials are tightly regulated by the federal government and must adhere to a comprehensive plan that must be approved by the Institutional Review Board (IRB). This board makes sure the study will not expose the participants to unethical practices or extreme risks.

All patients must be given detailed information about the study before they decide if they want to participate, including information about the treatments, any tests, and possible risks and benefits. Everything should be explained by a medical professional. Individuals who decide to participate in a study must sign an informed consent form, indicating that they have been presented with the information and that they understand it. (For patients who have been deemed unable to make such decisions, consent may be given by the patient's power of attorney.) Individuals should know that participants can choose to leave a study at any time.

Not everyone who wants to participate in a clinical trial is eligible. Each trial has its own entry criteria; for example, some choose only men, others only women, and some both; there are often age limitations; the extent of dementia may be a factor; and some exclude individuals who are taking specific medications or who have other medical conditions. Your doctor will discuss the criteria with you for any trial in which you are interested.

More Information

The Alzheimer's Disease Education and Referral Center (ADEAR) is an excellent resource for information about clinical trials for Alzheimer's disease; it includes a database of the trials currently in progress and which ones are actively recruiting patients. The ADEAR is a service of the National Institute on Aging (NIA), and the database is a joint project of the Food and Drug Administration and the NIA. The ADEAR can be reached at PO Box 8250, Silver Spring, MD 20907-8250, or online at www.alzheimers.org/adear, by telephone at 800-438-4380, or by e-mail at adear@alzheimers.org.

THE BOTTOM LINE

Medications, when used responsibly, can help individuals with Alzheimer's disease maintain independence, a good quality of life, and a sense of well-being. "Responsibly" means that patients, their medications, and their response to them should be reviewed regularly, preferably every two months, or more often if there are changes in the patient's behavior, needs, or health. Such vigilance helps provide patients and their caregivers the best quality of life possible.

Chapter 8

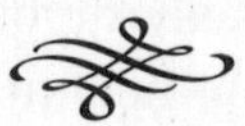

Complementary and Hormone Therapies

One of the rewarding things about working with people who have Alzheimer's disease is being able to say to patients and their caregivers, "Yes, there are drugs that can help you, but there are also some wonderful nondrug therapies we can try. These therapies can be used safely along with drugs, as needed, and they can greatly enhance your quality of life." Many patients and families are surprised by these words, but my experience shows them to be true. That is why I typically prescribe or recommend various herbal, nutritional, and hormonal therapies to my patients. And I suggest you work with your doctor to decide which of these therapies would be best for you.

A statement I have made several times throughout this book—that what's good for the heart is also good for the brain, and thus for Alzheimer's disease—holds true for complementary therapies as well. Because our arsenal of pharmaceutical substances for the treatment of Alzheimer's disease is not extensive, I am pleased that there are several natural, complementary treatments that have withstood the test of scientific research in the areas of memory loss and dementia and continue to be effective ways to help many patients.

Complementary therapy was "a real lifesaver," according to Maggie, who is caring for her eighty-eight-year-old mother, Ariel, who has Alzheimer's disease. Ariel moved into Maggie's home and was provided with her own apartment that is attached to the main house. Ariel, who has always been a gentle, soft-spoken woman, became irritable and restless shortly after moving in with her daughter. "She had insomnia, which kept me and my husband up all night, because we were worried that she might wander off or fall and injure herself," says Maggie. "Then, because she wasn't sleeping at night, she was irritable and drowsy during the day.

"My husband and I both work, and we need our sleep," says Maggie. "We thought of asking for sleeping pills, and we also talked about hiring someone to stay with her, day and night." Before taking these steps, Maggie called me and I suggested we give Ariel melatonin, a hormone that helps regulate the sleep-wake cycle. Although it isn't effective in all patients, it was the right choice for Ariel. Now she sleeps all night, and so do Maggie and her husband.

In this chapter we explore hormonal and complementary remedies that are showing promising signs in research, clinical trials, and anecdotal accounts. In another category are remedies that I believe are not helpful for people with Alzheimer's but which some individuals are using. Because many people have questions about these unproven remedies, I discuss these approaches as well and give you my reasons for not including them in my treatment plans.

BEST BETS

Estrogen

I am a strong advocate of prescribing biologically available estrogen (estradiol, the main type of estrogen made by the ovaries) for some but not all women who are at risk for Alzheimer's disease. Declining levels of estrogen have a negative impact on language skills, mood, concentration, attention, and other aspects of memory. Therefore, in my opinion, boosting those hormone levels can result in a significant improvement in cognitive functioning.

Estrogen and memory. Experts can see evidence of estrogen's role in memory and cognitive functioning in the brain because they have identified docking sites—places where estrogen attaches itself to brain tissue, including the hippocampus. The presence of these sites indicates that the hormone has tasks to perform in these areas. Estrogen may also increase the levels of major neurotransmitters in the brain that are involved in cognitive and behavioral functioning: acetylcholine (memory), dopamine (motor coordination), noradrenaline (mood), and serotonin (mood).

As I discussed in the chapter on prevention (chapter 5), estrogen replacement therapy should not be prescribed arbitrarily. Each woman's personal and family history needs to be considered before estrogen is recommended, because of the increased risks of certain cancers and the incidence of side effects. **The use of natural, soy-based estrogens (and micronized progesterone to balance the estrogen) is, I believe, the safest, most effective approach and the one I use with my patients, and with good results.**

Natural hormones. What's so special about natural hormones? They are obtained from substances called sterol analogues, which are derived primarily from soybeans (some also come from yams). These estrogen-like compounds are transformed in the laboratory to human bioidentical natural hormones. That means they are not foreign to the body, as are the horse urine–based hormones that were traditionally prescribed and which were used in many clinical studies. Thus natural hormones are easily accepted and used by the body. *Micronized* hormones have been broken down into tiny particles that allow them to be evenly and steadily absorbed by the body. Natural hormones work *with* the body, not against it. (For more information on natural hormones, see the books listed in "References and Suggested Readings.")

Prescribing estrogen. The needs of each woman must be evaluated individually before soy-based estrogens and micronized progesterone can be prescribed. Hormone therapies that are horse urine–based (e.g., Prempro, Premarin) are beneficial in some patients, but soy-based estrogens (e.g., Estrace, Climara) and combination hormone therapies (e.g., Femhrt) are beneficial in many more patients. Talk to your physician about these and other natural hormones. Natural hormones are available by prescription from your doctor and can be obtained from compounding pharmacies, which can prepare the hormones specifically for your needs. Your doctor can recommend compounding pharmacies that can meet your hormone requirements.

Folic Acid, Vitamin B_{12}, and Riboflavin

Although many people associate low levels of folic acid with an increased risk of birth defects, insufficient amounts of this B vitamin have also been linked with a greater risk of brain shrinkage in the elderly, a phenomenon that occurs in Alzheimer's disease.

The main benefit of maintaining a sufficient level of folic

acid may well be its ability to protect the brain from the toxic effects of homocysteine (see chapter 5), an amino acid that damages brain cells. To provide this protection, folic acid needs the assistance of another B vitamin, B_{12}, and evidence is pointing to the benefits of a third B vitamin, riboflavin, as well. All three of these B vitamins individually act as antioxidants and thus protect the nerve cells from oxidative damage, and it is believed that a combination of all three will be especially beneficial. A large-scale study is looking into this possibility now (see chapter 13, "The Future of Alzheimer's Disease").

Prescribing folic acid, vitamin B_{12}, and Riboflavin. I recommend that my patients take 1,000 mcg vitamin B_{12}, 1 mg folic acid, and 50 mg riboflavin daily. This combination does not come in one supplement, so three separate tablets need to be taken. For people who have mild cognitive impairment as well as high levels of homocysteine, I often prescribe injections of B_{12} and folic acid, as needed, until their homocysteine levels decline. Even though there is no definitive proof that this more aggressive approach will reduce the risk of mild cognitive impairment developing into Alzheimer's disease, I believe the research supports the effort and that individuals deserve to be given this risk-free and drug-free chance to reduce their risk.

Vitamin E

Results of a landmark, two-year clinical trial that tested vitamin E and selegiline (the MAO-B inhibitor I discussed in chapter 7) for their ability to slow the progression of Alzheimer's disease found that vitamin E may slow symptoms and functional signs of the disease by about seven months in people who have moderately severe Alzheimer's disease. This means that vitamin E can help patients retain their independence (e.g., the ability to perform daily activities such as bathing, eating, and dressing) for about seven months longer than people who do not take vitamin E. Thus the use of vitamin E can also help delay placement of individuals into nursing facilities. This delay not only allows patients and their families to spend more time together at home, it also gives caregivers more time to make nursing home or other care arrangements, should they be needed. The study did not, however, show vitamin E to cause any improvement in memory, attention, or language.

The study, published in the *New England Journal of Medicine* (1997), was significant because it gave physicians another treatment option, and one that is natural and with fewer side effects. (The drug selegiline was also found to delay disease progression, but it is associated with more expense and side effects; see chapter 7 for more information.) The fact that this powerful antioxidant benefits people who have Alzheimer's disease supports the idea that free radical damage of brain cells is involved in the disease and that vitamin E helps reduce that damage, at least for a while.

Prescribing vitamin E. Not all experts agree on the dose of vitamin E that is most effective in fighting advancement of the disease, but I find that 2,000 IU daily (the same amount used in the above-mentioned study) is optimal for my patients. No one should ever take this amount of vitamin E—or even smaller amounts—without a doctor's supervision, as this vitamin can cause gastrointestinal problems or bleeding in rare cases, and it can react negatively with some medications.

Ginkgo Biloba

For several years, I have encouraged my patients to use ginkgo biloba for its ability to improve memory and overall cognitive function for people who have dementia. This herb, which has been a mainstay of Chinese medicine for more than a thousand years, has been used in Europe for memory and concentration problems, depression, and anxiety for decades. It is rapidly gaining acceptance in the United States for the same purposes.

Although information about ginkgo's healing powers for people with dementia have trickled in over recent years, the largest comprehensive review of the herb's use in dementia to date was completed in October 2002. In the report of the study, which was conducted by the Alzheimer's Society and the Cochrane Collaboration, the investigators evaluated thirty-three clinical trials of ginkgo and concluded that there is strong evidence that the herb does indeed improve cognition and likely slows the degenerative process, without the risk of excess side effects.

The ingredients that appear to be behind ginkgo's benefits are flavonoids, natural substances that act as antioxidants. These flavonoids seem to enhance blood circulation in the brain, help more oxygen to reach the neurons, improve communication between nerve cells, and prevent the formation of blood clots. For many people who take ginkgo, these benefits result in better concentration and memory, improved mood, and less confusion.

Because ginkgo has blood-thinning properties, it should only be taken under a doctor's supervision, especially if your loved one is taking any other blood-thinning substances, such as aspirin or coumadin.

Prescribing ginkgo biloba. Typically I prescribe 120 to 240 mg daily, an amount that has been proven to be effective and safe. Because the bioavailability of American standardized preparations of this herb varies from brand to brand and within the same brand, I insist that patients obtain their supply from a German or Italian source where the preparation of this herb is well regulated.

Melatonin

When I have patients with Alzheimer's disease who are experiencing restlessness or mild insomnia, I find that supplementation with melatonin is helpful for some of them. A change in the circadian sleep-wake cycle due to the effects of aging and of disease is thought to be responsible. Caregivers like the fact that melatonin is not associated with the side effects that can accompany use of pharmaceutical sleeping aids (see chapter 7).

Melatonin is a hormone produced by the pineal gland, which is located in the center of the brain. Normally melatonin is secreted at night and acts as a sleep aid by improving sleep patterns and helping provide deep, restful sleep. In doses of between 3 and 9 mg a day, it has been shown to be beneficial as a sleep aid for up to three years in one study. However, a placebo-controlled trial of melatonin in Alzheimer's disease found it to be of little benefit for treating insomnia. Despite this, I find that some patients do benefit from this relatively innocuous drug, and I try this before moving on to other medications.

Prescribing melatonin. Dosing of melatonin is individual and should always be done under a doctor's supervision. Melatonin is available in regular pills, time-release tablets or capsules, sublingual lozenges, and sublingual liquid. The time-release products can provide the most consistent sleep.

UNCERTAIN OR UNPROVEN BENEFIT

Phosphatidylserine

Phosphatidylserine is a fatty substance that occurs naturally in the body. Its main tasks in the brain are to help maintain healthy nerve impulses and synapses, and to accumulate, store, and release neurotransmitters. These functions tend to decline with age, thus it has been suggested that supplementation with phosphatidylserine may enhance cognitive functions and improve mental ability.

Several clinical trials have looked at the benefits of phosphatidylserine in people who have Alzheimer's disease, and although improvements in memory and activities of daily living were seen in some patients, the findings are not convincing enough for me to prescribe this supplement. When patients come to me and say they are using phosphatidylserine or they ask me if they should take it, I tell them that while I see no harm in taking it, I'm not impressed with the research.

Acetyl-L-Carnitine

Acetyl-L-carnitine is a derivative of L-carnitine, a compound that is made in the body from the amino acids lysine and methionine. Unlike its cousin L-carnitine, which is promoted as a supplement to support heart function, acetyl-L-carnitine is used to protect brain and nerve cells.

According to several studies, acetyl-L-carnitine reduces free-radical damage in the brain and increases the production and levels of acetylcholine, the neurotransmitter that is in short supply in people who have Alzheimer's disease. Thus, in theory, acetyl-L-carnitine could help slow progression of Alzheimer's disease by preserving brain cells and boosting levels of acetylcholine. Based on available research, however, I am not convinced that acetyl-L-carnitine provides sufficient benefits for my patients. If individuals want to take acetyl-L-carnitine or are already taking it, I share what I know about the supplement and support their use if they decide to continue with it.

DHEA

Dehydroepiandrosterone (DHEA) is a hormone produced primarily by the adrenal glands, with smaller amounts made in the brain, ovaries, and testicles. DHEA leaves the adrenal glands and enters the bloodstream, where it is transformed into estrogens and testosterone.

Levels of DHEA decline as we age, and so this hormone has been the target of researchers who believe that restoring faltering DHEA levels will boost energy, improve mood, and enhance sex drive. Because DHEA is a precursor to estrogen and declining estrogen levels are associated with memory loss and other cognitive problems, some people who have Alzheimer's disease or memory problems take DHEA to reap the benefits of estrogen.

Although I do not prescribe DHEA to my patients, I work with those who have decided to take this hormone on their own. DHEA is a potent hormone, and I urge individuals to have their doctor monitor their use. Starting doses are often 5 mg daily, but even at this level or lower, some people experience adverse reactions. Women especially can develop hair growth in unwanted places, such as the face and chin, while, paradoxically, they experience hair loss from the scalp. Acne can occur at doses as low as 2 mg daily. Higher doses (typically 20 mg or more) can cause heart palpitations, menstrual irregularities, irritability, aggressiveness, headache, mood changes, and nervousness.

Choline and Lecithin

We know that insufficient levels of acetylcholine are a cause of memory problems and cognitive impairment, so one goal of treatment is to somehow reach and maintain adequate levels of this chemical. Two natural substances that are precursors of acetylcholine—choline and lecithin—have the ability to raise the levels of acetylcholine in the brain and enhance its production. Unfortunately, studies of its use in people who have Alzheimer's disease have not been promising. A few studies have shown some mild improvement in alertness and concentration, while others have demonstrated no benefits.

The lack of convincing improvement, along with side effects that include nausea, diarrhea, and irritability (associated with both choline and lecithin), plus incontinence, stomach pain, a fishy odor of the breath and in sweat (choline), and dry mouth (lecithin), make these two substances unacceptable treatment candidates. I advise people who are taking one or both of these supplements to stop treatment.

Huperzine A

Huperzine A is an extract derived from a type of moss (*Huperzia serrata*) and is a commonly used herb in Chinese medicine. Studies have shown that it has the ability to prevent the breakdown of acetylcholine, the substance in the brain that is involved in memory and learning. Because Alzheimer's disease is a condition characterized by low levels of acetylcholine, an agent that helps keep those levels up can be of benefit.

Most of the studies have been in animals and show that the herb can improve memory skills in older animals and in young animals in whom memory has been intentionally impaired. Studies in humans, all of which have been done in China, suggest huperzine A improves memory, cognition, and behavior in people who have Alzheimer's disease or other types of dementia, with only mild dizziness seen infrequently as a side effect. In one of those studies (double-blind, placebo-controlled), 58 percent of people with Alzheimer's disease showed improvement in these three areas, while only 36 percent of patients who took a placebo had improvement.

Huperzine A may hold some promise in the treatment of Alzheimer's disease, but I recommend that patients wait until more convincing findings are reported before trying this remedy.

Bacopa

Bacopa is an Ayurvedic medicinal herb traditionally used throughout India for over a thousand years to enhance memory. The use of bacopa has spread to the United States and other countries as well, and several scientific studies have been conducted in an attempt to identify whether it is effective.

Most of the studies of bacopa have been done in animals and have shown an improvement in learning skills. Of the few studies done in humans, one of the most recent was done in Australia in 2002. In this double-blind, placebo-controlled study, 76 adults ages forty to sixty-five had various memory functions tested before, during, and after the three-month trial. Bacopa significantly improved the ability to retain new information; however, attention, verbal and visual short-term memory, and anxiety were not improved. No side effects have been reported.

Although bacopa may have some potential as a complementary remedy for cognitive functioning, I would not recommend its use until more research has been done.

THE BOTTOM LINE

I believe the use of complementary remedies for the treatment of Alzheimer's disease and its associated symptoms can make a significant difference in the lives of people who live with this form of dementia, as well as those of their caregivers. If you have a physician who is not using any of these approaches, I encourage you to raise the subject with him or her. You may also want to get a second opinion from another doctor who has knowledge of complementary methods. I believe such steps are important because both your loved one and you deserve to have access to as many effective and promising treatments as possible.

Chapter 9

Stimulating the Senses

A garden of blooming flowers. The sweetness of a chocolate-dipped ice cream cone. The softness of a Persian cat's fur. The melodious sound of a symphony. All of these are examples of things that stimulate the senses and can bring pleasure to those who experience them. But these sensory pleasures are much more than ways to brighten our days: they can also be a joyful, drug-free way to help improve the quality of life of a person who has Alzheimer's disease.

For people who have Alzheimer's disease, life can often be confusing, frustrating, and frightening—negative feelings that caregivers are often desperate to relieve. These negative feelings can cause or contribute to behavioral and psychological problems, which are a source of much distress for both patients and their caregivers. In fact, behavioral problems such as wandering and aggression are among the main reasons caregivers place their loved ones in a nursing or other care facility, as these actions can be not only difficult to deal with but also harmful to the patients and those around them.

The good news is that these symptoms are responsive to treatment, not just with medications, which I prefer to use after I've tried other approaches, but with nondrug methods. Along with complementary therapies, which we discussed in the last chapter, other nonpharmaceutical approaches include those that stimulate and please the senses—things caregivers and families can try at home to help improve the quality of life of their loved ones.

Seventy-nine-year-old Stella is proof that this approach can work. Stella lived with her daughter, Constance, and her family in the suburbs. When Stella's irritability and aggressive behavior (she would slap people when she got agitated) got to be more than she could tolerate, Constance contemplated moving her mother into a nursing home. On a whim, a cousin visited Stella and Constance and brought her black Lab mix along. Stella showed a great interest in the dog and her disposition improved when the dog was there. After the dog visited several more times, Constance noticed that her mother's mood and behavior improved significantly in the dog's presence. Constance went to the local humane society, found a beautiful black Lab–collie mix named Molly (I find that mixed breeds have superior temperaments to those of purebreds and thus are preferable as companions for people who have Alzheimer's disease), and brought her home. Now Stella and Molly are inseparable, and Stella's attitude and behavior are much improved. There are now several studies that support a role for dogs in reducing agitation in Alzheimer's.

Naturally, if your loved one is displaying behavioral and psychological problems you should first have him or her seen by a specialist in this area, who may want to prescribe medications. However, I believe it's important for patients and families to know that other treatment approaches can be effective as well, and they may want to try them first. And even though most of the therapies discussed in this chapter have not been the subject of clinical trials, patients and caregivers alike can attest to their success.

USING ART

When Helen is working with watercolors, she sits and smiles at everyone. And this is a big change from the way she usually acts. "I never knew she would be interested in painting," says Amy of her eighty-year-old mother, who was diagnosed with Alzheimer's disease six years ago. "But when she's at the adult center for art therapy or she's at home painting, she's a different person. She's much less agitated, she doesn't argue with me and my husband, and she doesn't shout. I let her paint as much as she wants."

Art therapy is a way people can express themselves through work with paint, charcoal, clay, paper, or other media. It's been shown that expression through art is an effective way to reduce depression, release stress, and enhance self-esteem. Creating art can also improve hand-eye coordination and stimulate neurological activity in the brain. Therapists who introduce art projects to patients with dementia find that the individuals are more relaxed and sociable and are less depressed than patients who don't do art therapy. In fact, studies show that heart rate and respiration rate slow down and blood pressure decreases when people are involved in an activity they enjoy.

Art therapy has proved so successful that the Alzheimer's Association has instituted a project called "Memories in the Making Art Program." The program, which originated in Orange County, California, provides art materials, instruction, and supervision for people who have Alzheimer's disease. Participants are allowed to try painting and drawing, even if they've never done either one before. Many other local chapters of the Alzheimer's Association have instituted the program as well. You can contact your local Alzheimer's Association chapter to see if "Memories in the Making" is available in your area (see the Appendix).

One reason art therapy is so effective may be that it allows individuals to release pent-up emotions—feelings they are unable to express verbally. Creating art is an opportunity for people to illustrate their fears and anger, as well as leave lasting mementos of their feelings.

If you'd like to introduce art activities to your loved one, consider the following tips:

- See if there is a creative program for people with dementia offered in your area. Contact the local chapter of the Alzheimer's Association or talk to a social worker or therapist at your local hospital about any ongoing programs.
- If your loved one is not able or ready to create art, he or she may enjoy going to an art museum or looking at art books, which you can borrow from the library.
- Consider playing soothing music in the background during art sessions. This can enhance the creative experience and reduce anxiety.
- It's not important for the individuals to "complete" a piece of art. Art therapy is about the creative process, not the end result. Whatever your loved one creates is perfect the way it is, because it is an act of healing.
- Keep the project on an adult level; that is, don't offer patients crayons (unless they prefer them), construction paper, or felt markers, as many people associate these with children. People with Alzheimer's disease who think they are being treated like a child may act out. Allow patients to use watercolors, charcoal, clay, or pastels; an easel adds a nice touch.

- Always consider safety. Avoid sharp tools and toxic substances.
- Do not criticize the art that is created. If your loved one paints a green sky, that's the way he or she wants it to be.

USING MUSIC AND DANCE

The author and neurologist Oliver Sacks once said that he regarded "music therapy as a tool of great power in many neurological disorders," including Alzheimer's disease, because it has the "unique capacity to organize or reorganize cerebral function when it has been damaged." Research certainly backs up Dr. Sacks's statement. In one study conducted by the University of Miami, a month-long program of music therapy (30 to 40 minutes of therapy five days a week for one month) improved the sleeping difficulties and behavior of people with Alzheimer's disease by stimulating higher production of melatonin, a hormone known to help promote calm in different areas of the brain. Music therapy also raised the levels of two other hormones that can influence mood—norepinephrine and epinephrine—but the levels of these hormones didn't stay elevated six weeks after the therapy was discontinued. The levels of melatonin, however, did remain high.

The secret is to choose music or tunes the individual *knows* and *enjoys*. Classical music, soft jazz, big band, folk songs, even environmental sounds (waterfalls, forest sounds, ocean waves), hard rock, and pop songs can have a calming effect. In some individuals, music therapy may reduce the need for sedating medications.

Marilyn saw a significant difference in her mother's behavior once she introduced music into the house. "She had always enjoyed show tunes," says Marilyn of her seventy-nine-year-old mother. "Mother was living with us, and her behavior was becoming more and more disruptive. We didn't want to place her in a nursing home yet, so the doctor suggested music therapy. We began playing old show tunes on CDs all day long. The change in her behavior was almost immediate. She was much less aggressive, she slept better at night, and she didn't wander nearly as much. We were able to keep her at home for nearly another year before her health deteriorated and we had to place her in a nursing facility. But we got the gift of that year. Now we keep a CD player in her room at the nursing home, and the nurses say it still helps keep her more calm." In my office, where we often play old standards, we've had mute, unresponsive patients hum and sometimes sing along with songs.

What makes music such a powerful force? Music has several elements—pitch, accent, timbre, melody, rhythm—that are processed in different parts of the brain, although it arouses us at a very basic level—the brain stem. Language, however, is processed in only one place in the brain—the back of the left temporal lobe. Therefore, people who have problems processing language can still appreciate music, at least at the most primitive level. That's why people who have severe dementia can still respond to music, because they are reacting from their brain stem. Thus music therapy can be useful with people who are at all stages of Alzheimer's disease.

Music even helps those who seemingly have lost or nearly lost the ability to speak. Some people with Alzheimer's will sing along with a song they remember from years ago, yet they rarely speak at any other time. Even when the music stops, they will often continue to sing or hum the song, proof that music has the ability to reach deep within the memory centers in the brain.

If you haven't tried music therapy, you might consider adding it to your loved one's life.

- Choose music they once enjoyed, or if you don't know their musical taste, try tunes popular when he or she was in their teens or twenties.
- Introduce background music during bathing, meals, or any other time he or she is especially agitated or restless and see what effect it has. You may find that it has a soothing effect on you as well!
- Use tapes or CDs, as these provide continuous music. Radio programs have too many interruptions, which can cause confusion.
- Eliminate competing sounds. Turn off the television or radio, and close windows and doors if there are other sounds that can be disturbing or disruptive.
- When appropriate, encourage your loved one to sing along, clap to the music, or even dance.
- I often recommend that dance be used for those patients who will not comply with physical therapy. This keeps them limber and joyful. Lucille is a seventy-two-year-old retired nurse who became very reluctant to keep active, either with walking or exercises recommended by her doctor, even though she is physically able to do so. Her daughter, Sharon, remembered how much her mother used to enjoy dancing with her now deceased husband. So Sharon gathered together some ballroom dance CDs and enlisted the help of her uncle, Edgar, who also loves to dance. Now Lucille not only enjoys dancing at home once a week with Edgar, but Sharon and Edgar take her to a senior center once a week for dancing as well. Some patients with difficulty walking also benefit from dance.

USING HORTICULTURE

There's something about nature, the beauty and mystery of growing plants, that seems to calm many individuals who have Alzheimer's disease.

When patients work with plants, they direct their focus outside themselves, and this tends to reduce inappropriate behavior. Putting their hands into dirt, planting seeds, transplanting seedlings, picking weeds from a garden, watering plants, decorating pots, and arranging flowers are all activities that stimulate the senses, improve hand-eye coordination, promote physical activity, and build self-confidence. People who plant seeds, wait for them to sprout, and then watch them grow into viable plants can have a sense of purpose and feel needed.

Stanley, a seventy-seven-year-old retired factory worker, certainly fits that picture. During his younger years, he had spent his spare time tending a very large vegetable garden and several flower beds in his yard. Now, in his fifth year of Alzheimer's disease, he spends hours each day on the back patio, hovering over several dozen pots of geraniums and pansies and flats of various vegetable plants that he eventually transplants into the yard.

"He lives for those plants," says his wife, Christine. "They're the first thing he looks for in the morning. Sometimes he spends hours just walking up and down looking at the plants. He's safe and happy, and that makes me happy."

You don't need a lot of room to introduce a few plants into the life of a person who has Alzheimer's disease. You can begin with several potted plants on the patio or a windowsill, or lined up on a table placed against a sunny window. If you have space in your yard and it is a safe, secure environment, you might start a flower or vegetable bed. Individuals who have difficulty bending down or kneeling on the ground may want to work with potted plants or flats set on a table. Special gardening instruments, referred to as "enabling tools," are available from many garden supply centers. These items reduce the strain placed on weak arms, arthritic knees, and sore wrists.

USING TOUCH

Touch is a powerful, intimate, nonverbal form of communication that has the ability to heal in many ways. Several studies, including one at the University of Texas, have found that slow, gentle massage on people who have Alzheimer's disease can significantly reduce pacing, aggression, wandering, anxiety, and insomnia. In some cases, it can reduce a patient's need for sedating medications. Massage can also improve blood circulation and ease muscle aches and pains.

Although touch is a universal way to communicate, some people don't like to be touched because it brings up bad memories. A person who was physically abused in the past, for example, may be frightened by any attempt at massage, and so you should not pursue it any further.

If, however, your loved one is receptive to massage, remember to apply minimal pressure. Forget the typical picture of massage—chopping motions, kneading, and slapping are not to be used with people who have Alzheimer's disease.

Depending on the temperament of your loved one, you may begin by simply gently massaging the hands or feet. You can use lotion if desired (perhaps scented with one of the essential oils we discuss later in this chapter under "Stimulating Smell"). A 10-minute massage daily, perhaps after dinner and before bedtime, can be very relaxing and help the individual sleep. Always be flexible, however. Accept the fact that after giving your loved one a massage for many days, he or she may one day, without warning, not want to be touched. Forgo the massage for that day, but do offer it again another day.

The benefit of massage that can't be measured is the caring and compassion you convey to your loved one during the massage. Touch is an intimate activity that communicates without words. And because your loved one may not be able to understand your words, chances are good that your love is being communicated through your touch.

Reflexology is a hands-on therapy that is based on the concept that each part of the body—organs, glands, and structures—has a corresponding point on the feet. Each point on the foot is believed to be linked to the corresponding body part via an energy channel called a meridian. When various points on the feet are stimulated (pressed or massaged with the fingers), it prompts the release of energy along the meridians, which allows the corresponding body part to function more naturally.

One reason reflexology may have a calming effect is that the stimulation of the nerve endings (there are 7,200 in the feet), blood vessels, and muscles releases endorphins (the body's natural painkilling chemicals), increases blood circulation to the tissues, and improves the transport of nutrients and oxygen to the cells. Some people say having a reflexology session is like having your entire body massaged.

THE USE OF PETS

For people with Alzheimer's disease who once had pets or who love animals, pet therapy can be an effective and joyful way to enhance their lives. It's a wonderful feeling to see the faces of my patients light up when they are in the presence of a beautiful black Labrador or a purring tabby cat. Countless studies have shown that pets have the ability to reduce blood pressure, heart rate, and respiration rate; they improve behavior, stimulate the senses, help bring up memories, alleviate loneliness, enhance mood, increase communication, and give people a sense of purpose. Pets can offer unconditional love, and this feeling alone can make a tremendous difference in the lives of people who are living with feelings of frustration, anger, and fear.

Pet therapy can be considered on several levels, depending on the status of your loved one and the part you play in his or her care. If you are caring for a loved one at home and there are pets already there, you have an opportunity to see how they interact and if the responses are positive. If no pets are currently accessible to your loved one, bringing one into the home is an option, but you must consider whether you will have the time to care for the animal and for all the responsibilities that go along with pet ownership. For some families, this added burden is too much.

Another option is to have a friend or family member visit with his or her pet—as long as the animal is gentle and compatible with your loved one. Colette is a seventy-one-year-old grandmother of three who was diagnosed with Alzheimer's disease three years ago. She lives in an apartment downstairs from her daughter, Suzanne, who keeps an eye on her mother but lets her maintain her independence as much as possible. Suzanne noticed that her mother was becoming more and more withdrawn and didn't want to socialize. Suzanne works full-time and so can't spend time with her mother during the day.

"I was concerned that she wasn't getting enough stimulation during the day," says Suzanne. "She's content to sit in front of the television. But Mom has always liked dogs, and our neighbor has a golden retriever mix that she walks every morning. So I asked her if she would bring her dog over for a visit with my mother several times a week. And she offered to do even more than that; she said she'd take my mother along on her walks. Now my mother looks forward to walking with the dog. True, she pays more attention to the dog than she does our neighbor, but her mood has improved and she's getting exercise. I can't thank my neighbor and her dog enough."

For some people, the best alternative to having a pet already in the home is to utilize the pet therapy sessions at an adult day care center for people who have Alzheimer's disease. You can check with your local Alzheimer's Association chapter to see if such sessions are available in your area.

If your loved one is in a nursing facility and pet therapy is part of the program they provide, encourage his or her participation. These sessions, as well as those at adult day care centers, are usually run by individuals who have been trained in handling pets for this purpose. The animals too have been specially screened for temperament and energy level. In addition to cats and dogs, rabbits, birds, ferrets, and pot-bellied pigs may be part of the program. Some nursing facilities even contract with local zoos and have more exotic animals brought in to see the residents.

If you do introduce a pet into the life of a person who has Alzheimer's disease, remember to match the animal's size, temperament, and energy level with that of your loved one. A dog can encourage your loved one to be physically active (walking the dog, playing catch) as well as provide companionship and a feeling of security. If the person with Alzheimer's is frightened by a dog or cat, perhaps the company of a confined animal such as a bird, hamster, or fish may be soothing. Some people can spend hours watching tropical fish swim in a tank. Others enjoy talking to a parrot or parakeet or observing the antics of hamsters or gerbils playing in a cage.

Recently I began to bring my two Great American Mutts to the office, and they break the ice right away when patients come to see me. It's heartwarming to see how patients and their families respond to the dogs. They greatly reduce agitation in my anxious patients. The staff, myself included, are happier, too.

STIMULATING SMELL

Aromatherapy is the use of essential oils (the essences from various parts of plants) to support healing, through inhalation and/or application to the skin. If you doubt the power that smells can have over you, think about some memorable events or situations in your past: big family dinners, a vacation at the beach, the night your husband proposed at your favorite Italian restaurant. Can you smell hot apple pie, the salty surf, or garlic and oregano without thinking of those times? That's because there is a powerful link between the olfactory nerves (responsible for smell) and memory. The memories of different smells are stored in the limbic section of the brain, the area that is involved with memory and emotions. Different smells are associated with different memories, so when you smell a certain aroma, say, apple pie, it may stimulate a memory of your grandmother. Although there's no evidence that aromatherapy can improve memory, the use of essential oils may improve behavior and reduce anxiety and stress in some people.

Among the dozens of essential oils available, those typically used in nursing facilities and hospitals to help soothe patients and improve mood are sweet orange, lavender, eucalyptus, and peppermint. These are among the most soothing, uplifting, and anti-anxiety oils available. You can use these same oils at home in any of the various ways described below. There's an added benefit: these oils also help calm the nerves of caregivers as well!

Essential oils are typically available in small (1 ounce or less) opaque glass containers and can be purchased from some large department stores, health food stores, candle or herb shops, gift shops, by mail order, and on the Internet. Look for oils that say "100 percent pure."

Ways to Use Aromatherapy

Depending on the preferences of your loved one, you can introduce essential oils in many different ways:

- Place about 20 drops in bath water and swirl the water to mix them in.
- Use essential oils as massage oils. Not everyone likes to be touched or massaged, but if your loved one is amenable to a hand or foot massage, lotions scented with essential oils rubbed into the hands or feet can be very soothing.
- Place 5 to 10 drops in the water in a humidifier. You can leave the humidifier on during the day or at night, when it may help your loved one sleep.
- Add 5 to 10 drops to 2 ounces of distilled water in a mister and spritz the air in the room.
- Light oil-scented candles.
- Place a few drops on a handkerchief or tissue and inhale gently.
- Add essential oils to an electric or terra-cotta aromatherapy lamp or diffuser, which are available from specialty shops.

Aromatherapy Do's and Don'ts

- Before you use any essential oil on the skin, you must dilute it. Essential oils are very potent and can irritate the skin. Choose a carrier oil (e.g., sunflower, almond, jojoba, walnut) and mix 5 to 6 drops of the essential oil in 1 teaspoon of the carrier oil, and apply this mixture to the skin.
- Check for allergic reactions. Allergies to sweet orange, lavender, and eucalyptus are very rare; some people

do have a reaction to peppermint. To check for allergic reactions, mix 3 drops of the chosen essential oil with 1 teaspoon of a carrier oil. Rub a little of this mixture on your loved one in the crook of the arm, behind the ear, or inside the wrist. (You should do this for yourself as well if you will be handling the oils.) Leave the treated area uncovered and unwashed for 24 hours. If no redness or itching occurs, the oil is safe to use.

- Avoid using the oils where food is served or during meals. The aroma can interfere with the ability to taste, or the food smells could overpower the aroma of the oils.
- Essential oils are very potent and evaporate easily, so they should be stored in a dark, cool place and their tops should be kept on tightly at all times.

SNOEZELEN ROOMS

Imagine walking into a room that has been specially designed to cater to all or nearly all of your senses. You may hear the sound of water rushing along a stream, birds chirping, and the gentle rustle of leaves in the wind. On the walls you may see posters or projected pictures of fields, forests, waterfalls, and flower gardens. The air may be infused with the aroma of flowers, and around the room there may be inviting recliners, bean bag chairs, furry pillows, and vases full of silk flowers.

This is an example of a Snoezelen environment, a multisensory room where stimulating experiences, activities, and objects are offered to help individuals who are living with frustration, agitation, aggression, and loss of concentration and memory. Decades of using this approach, primarily in Europe but more recently in the United States, have shown that

Snoezelen rooms may help increase concentration, awareness, alertness, and calmness while at the same time decreasing agitation, depression, difficulties with communication, wandering behaviors, and aggression.

Snoezelen rooms have been created primarily in long-term nursing care facilities and in some adult day care centers in the United States. Rooms are typically designed around a specific theme, such as a flower garden, a tropical island, big band music, or an amusement park. The materials used to create the mood can vary greatly and are chosen with security and effectiveness in mind. Support staff should always be present in the room with patients to ensure their safety and comfort.

If you think your loved one would enjoy the experience of a Snoezelen room, you can call nursing homes or adult day care centers in your area to see if such rooms are available. Although not everyone who has Alzheimer's disease is receptive to a Snoezelen room experience, many do find great comfort in them. Caregivers and friends of people who have Alzheimer's disease also report that visiting their loved ones is much more relaxing and pleasant when they do so in Snoezelen rooms.

THE BOTTOM LINE

Therapies that engage the senses may have a calming, balancing effect on people who have Alzheimer's disease, as well as provide opportunities for caregivers to share quality time with their loved ones. Most of the approaches discussed in this chapter can easily be incorporated into an individual's lifestyle and enrich it in ways perhaps not verifiable in scientific research but evident in the smiles and pleasure they bring to the people who enjoy them.

Chapter 10

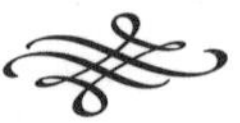

When Alzheimer's Isn't the Only Health Concern

Lillian had been diagnosed with Alzheimer's disease for nearly six years, and for the last two she had been living with her daughter, Rose, and Rose's husband, Tom. Although Lillian's short-term memory was poor, she seemed to be in good health otherwise. Generally she was in good spirits, and she enjoyed playing with her grandchildren and working in the garden. For much of her adult life she had been a few pounds overweight, and now, at seventy years of age, she was about fifteen pounds heavier than her ideal weight. Rose worried a little about her mother's weight, especially because Lillian loved to eat sweets, but she didn't want to "deprive my mother of the foods she loves."

When Rose noticed that her mother seemed unusually tired and that her usually pleasant disposition had deteriorated into crankiness, she attributed it to worsening Alzheimer's disease.

But when another family member mentioned that perhaps Lillian had diabetes, which runs in the family, Rose immediately took her mother to her doctor for a glucose tolerance test. Lillian tested positive for type II diabetes, and once her diet was modified and an oral diabetic medication was prescribed, her cheerful personality returned and so did her energy.

Lillian's case is not unusual in one sense: many people with Alzheimer's disease also live with one or more other medical ailments. Because Alzheimer's disease tends to affect older adults, major health problems common in this population, such as cardiovascular disease, urinary tract infections, diabetes, and Parkinson's disease, are frequently part of a patient's overall health condition. In fact, it is worth repeating here that many of the risk factors for Alzheimer's disease are the same as those for heart disease, stroke, and diabetes, so it is not uncommon for people who have Alzheimer's to have one or more of these conditions as well.

What *is* more unusual about Lillian's case is that something was done about it. I find that, sometimes, we physicians tend to be less aggressive not only in diagnosing these illnesses but in treating them as well, especially among people who are in a more advanced stage of Alzheimer's. The problem is, these other diseases can have a significant and detrimental effect not only on how Alzheimer's disease progresses but also on the individuals' quality of life, as well as that of their caregivers. That's why I believe it is critical to conscientiously treat these accompanying medical conditions.

Although identifying and treating major medical concerns is important, we must not forget health problems that may seem less critical (at least initially). People with advanced Alzheimer's disease often cannot communicate information to their caregivers about aches, pains, discomfort, or injuries; thus it is not uncommon for them to become agitated when they experience headache or migraine, constipation, bedsores, pneumonia, bruises, dental pain, stomach distress, and other health problems and be unable to let anyone know what's wrong.

In this chapter we bring to light the importance of identifying and treating those health issues that can accompany Alzheimer's disease in the hope of improving the lives of those who are challenged by them. We also give you some tips on how to recognize when your loved one may be experiencing these issues.

CARDIOVASCULAR CONDITIONS

Norman, an eighty-seven-year-old semiretired attorney, had been diagnosed with Alzheimer's disease for five years and at home was pursuing aggressive cognitive rehabilitation, which, along with medications, was allowing him to still see clients occasionally and keep up an active social life that included going to art exhibits, visiting friends, and dining out several times a week. When he suddenly began to experience episodes of lost balance, mental fogginess, and confusion, his first fear, and that of his wife and caregiver, Adrianne, was that his Alzheimer's disease was taking a turn for the worse. He saw his internist, who assured him that all was well. But Norman didn't feel well.

Norman came to my office and, because of the episodic nature of his symptoms and an irregular pulse, I suspected that something else besides Alzheimer's was responsible for his symptoms, so I encouraged him to see a cardiologist. The cardiologist uncovered an arrhythmia, or an irregular heartbeat. Norman had a pacemaker installed, and within a few weeks of surgery his cognitive abilities returned to their presurgery state, his confusion ended, and he had no more balance problems.

Norman's situation is a good example of how a medical condition that is seemingly unrelated to Alzheimer's disease can have a significant impact on it. Oftentimes, cardiac arrhythmias in particular go unrecognized in older adults, especially because they cause symptoms such as falls, fainting, and loss of balance, which are typically associated with aging. In Norman's case, and in that of many other patients I have seen over the years, prompt identification and treatment of arrhythmia made a significant difference in the progress of the Alzheimer's and in their quality of life.

If your loved one begins to show these or other uncharacteristic or sudden symptoms, please bring them to the attention of your physician immediately.

- Shortness of breath
- Frequent falls
- Fluttering of the heart or palpitations
- Dizziness
- Sweating accompanied by cold and clammy skin

Prompt recognition of a cardiovascular problem can help maintain a better quality of life for your loved one and perhaps can even save his or her life.

URINARY TRACT INFECTIONS

Urinary tract infections occur when bacteria are not adequately eliminated from the bladder or the urethra. These infections are common among older adults, especially women and individuals who are bedridden. They are a leading cause of death among people who have late-stage Alzheimer's disease, because the body is unable to effectively fight the infection.

Indications that your loved one may have a urinary tract infection include the following:

- Pain or burning when urinating
- Increased frequency of urination

- Increased agitation
- Feeling the need to urinate often
- Increased drowsiness
- Fever
- Blood in the urine
- Fatigue
- Increased confusion

For Abigail, the telltale signs were a sudden worsening of memory and unexpected drowsiness. At age eighty-nine, Abigail was still able to enjoy many of life's amenities, such as going to the symphony and visiting with friends. She had been diagnosed with Alzheimer's disease for nearly ten years, so when she suddenly experienced a dramatic increase in agitation and confusion, her family thought it was a dire sign. After she had been displaying these symptoms for about a week, her niece noticed blood in Abigail's urine and took her aunt to the doctor. The doctor ran a test, uncovered a urinary tract infection, and began treatment immediately. Abigail was back to her preinfection self in a matter of days, thanks to an observant family member and Abigail's physician.

Urinary tract infections can be treated with antibiotics, so you should contact your doctor immediately if you suspect an infection is present. To help prevent urinary tract infections, and to assist medical treatment should one occur, make sure your loved one drinks at least six to eight glasses of noncaffeinated, nonalcoholic liquids daily. Pure water and diluted (one part water to two parts juice) unsweetened cranberry juice are recommended as preventive and treatment measures for urinary tract infections. Also, monitor personal hygiene in those persons with advanced Alzheimer's.

DIABETES

It is estimated that about 20 million Americans have diabetes, yet *half of them don't know it.* That means about 10 million people are walking around with unacknowledged, untreated diabetes. Among people who have diabetes, the risk of getting Alzheimer's disease is nearly twice that of people who don't have diabetes. This risk increases to more than four times among individuals with diabetes who take insulin.

Signs and symptoms of diabetes may be overlooked by physicians and caregivers of people who have Alzheimer's disease. Indications of diabetes include the following:

- Blurry vision
- Tingling and/or numbness in the legs, feet, fingers, and hands
- Frequent skin, gum, and/or urinary tract infections
- Itchy skin and/or genitals
- Drowsiness
- Frequent urination
- Excessive thirst
- Fatigue
- Nausea and vomiting
- Mood changes
- Confusion

If your loved one has complained of or if you have noticed any of these signs, and he or she has not been tested for diabetes, I encourage you to do so. Recognition of symptoms may take some careful observation on your part, which is why I suggest you make notes for a few days. Proper control of blood sugar levels can greatly improve an individual's awareness, energy level, and mood, and thus enhance their life as well as yours.

PARKINSON'S DISEASE

Parkinson's disease is a neurological condition that affects more than 1.5 million Americans. In recent years, there has been increasing evidence of similarities between Alzheimer's disease and Parkinson's disease in both symptoms and the physical changes they cause in the body, including the presence of plaques and tangles in the brain. These findings have led some experts to say that these two diseases may be related, while others suggest that many people simply have these conditions at the same time.

Until we have more definitive research findings, it's safe to say that 20 to 30 percent of people who have Parkinson's disease also have symptoms of Alzheimer's disease. Unfortunately, symptoms of Parkinson's disease are routinely overlooked among people who have been diagnosed with Alzheimer's disease. Again, as with diabetes, I encourage caregivers to make notes of any changes in movement, gait, or activities to see if a pattern or trend develops. They could be an indication that something besides Alzheimer's disease is at work.

Symptoms of Parkinson's disease in people who have Alzheimer's disease can include the following:

- Problems with walking, including little or no arm swing, shuffling, freezing (temporarily being unable to initiate or continue with walking, especially in areas such as doorways), and difficulty making turns
- Rigidity, or stiffness, that can include a lack of facial expression
- A slow (pill-rolling) tremor (resting tremor of the thumb and fingers) of the hand when at rest
- Poor balance and easy tripping
- Slow movements

Symptoms of Parkinson's disease can be treated with medication, and regular physical activity has been shown to help slow progression of the disease. These steps can only be taken, however, if the disease is recognized and diagnosed. Bring any suspicions of or concerns about Parkinson's disease to the attention of your physician.

OTHER HEALTH ISSUES

Later in the course of the illness, your loved one may have a headache or stomach cramps, a bad bruise or a toothache, yet he or she can't verbally communicate the feeling to you. Yet you may suspect something is amiss if the person with Alzheimer's disease suddenly begins to display unusual behavior. Shouting or moaning, refusing to eat or drink, worsening mood, pushing people away, increased agitation or restlessness, or refusing to do activities he or she had been doing all along—these are some common indications that the individual is experiencing some type of discomfort or pain.

However, such behaviors can also indicate something besides a physical ailment, such as a reaction to medication, a response to something your loved one heard or saw, or a worsening of the disease. Thus to uncover whether there is a health issue, you may need to switch into "detective" mode. Rosalie and Irwin are an example.

Irwin's Story

For three days, Rosalie, a sixty-eight-year-old retired florist, was perplexed by her husband's sudden change in behavior. Irwin, a seventy-two-year-old retired machinist, usually was content to tinker in his workshop during the day, sit in the garden, and watch television. Although he tended to wander if

Rosalie didn't keep an eye on him, he was usually pleasant, ate whatever Rosalie made for him, and rarely raised his voice.

So when Irwin suddenly refused to eat, hid in his room, and shouted, "Splinters, splinters!" whenever Rosalie asked him what was wrong, she became concerned. "I thought he had gotten a splinter in his finger or his foot while in his workshop, but I couldn't see anything," says Rosalie. "And I couldn't understand what splinters had to do with his not wanting to eat." By the afternoon of the third day of this unusual behavior, Rosalie was very upset and didn't know where to turn. That afternoon, Irwin fell asleep in a recliner in the living room, and he slept with his mouth wide open.

"I don't know what made me think to look inside his mouth," says Rosalie, "but when I did, I noticed an abscess inside his mouth. Suddenly his refusing to eat and his odd behavior made sense.

"I guess 'splinters' to him meant something that hurt, and his mouth hurt," says Rosalie. She immediately took Irwin to a dentist, who found a serious infection; it was cleared up in a few days with medication. Within a week, Irwin was back in his workshop and eating again.

The following discussion of common medical issues among people with Alzheimer's disease explains the types of signals you may see, how to look for subtle indications of a problem, and tips on how to handle each situation. Alzheimer's disease can cause a wide range of behaviors and moods, therefore it isn't possible to predict how your loved one will act out any health problem or how he or she will respond to any of the suggestions offered here. However, the hints included in the following sections have helped many caregivers manage these health issues.

Constipation

Constipation can be a difficult problem to identify unless you make a point to regularly monitor your loved one's bowel habits. Symptoms of constipation can include stomach or intestinal pain or cramps, nausea, or headache, all of which may be impossible for individuals to communicate. You may notice behavioral changes, a refusal to eat, or postures that indicate pain in the intestinal area, such as hunching over or holding the arms crossed across the stomach.

Constipation can develop when individuals with Alzheimer's change their eating habits, perhaps refusing to eat certain foods (e.g., those high in fiber such as whole grains, vegetables, or beans) or refusing to eat at all. Sometimes constipation is a side effect of medication, so check with your doctor to see if the problem is a reaction to something your loved one is taking. Lack of physical exercise and generalized inactivity also are major factors in constipation.

If you discover constipation is the problem, the best approach may be a natural one: increase intake of fiber (e.g., encourage foods such as cooked carrots, oatmeal, oat bran muffins, winter squash, broccoli, dates, kidney beans, lima beans) and adequate liquids (six to eight glasses daily), along with use of a mild laxative. Consult your doctor about the type of laxative that is best to take. Most importantly, increase the amount of daily physical activity.

Dehydration

People who have Alzheimer's disease, like elderly persons in general, often do not drink as much liquid as they should, which can lead to dehydration. This can be especially troublesome if they have diabetes, a urinary tract infection (see discussion in this chapter), diarrhea, or if they have been vomiting. Indications that a loved one may be experiencing dehydration include:

- Increased confusion
- Dizziness
- Loss of balance when rising from a seated or lying position
- Rapid pulse
- Diarrhea or constipation

You want your loved one to drink enough fluids, and for those fluids to be healthy ones. Water, noncaffeinated, and nonsugary beverages are best—diluted fruit and vegetable juices (two parts water to one part juice) and herbal teas are preferred. Avoid beverages that contain caffeine in the evening because they can increase restlessness, anxiety, and sleeplessness.

Dental Problems

Toothaches, abscesses, cavities, poorly fitting dentures, gum disease, and other dental problems occur frequently among people who have Alzheimer's disease. This is partially due to less diligent brushing of teeth and partially due to medications that may dry one's mouth, as they reduce the antibacterial saliva in the mouth. Some patients display obvious signs of discomfort, such as holding their hand to their mouth or cheek or pointing to the painful area in their mouth. Others, like Irwin, may manifest behavior changes and refuse to eat, leaving you to wonder what could be wrong, if anything.

The best thing you can do is to be observant. Note whether your loved one grimaces or makes a face when eating or drinking. You can ask the individual to open his or her mouth wide for you, but some people refuse to do so. Don't force the issue.

If you suspect there is a dental problem, talk to a dentist who is used to working with people who have dementia. Before any procedures are done, tell the dentist about any medications the patient is taking.

You can help avoid dental problems by following these guidelines:

- Help your loved one to brush after every meal. If your efforts are resisted, suggest swishing with water or using mouth swabs. If these suggestions fail, encourage him or her to eat crunchy, raw vegetables or fruit at the end of a meal (e.g., fresh raw apples, carrots, cucumbers, pears). These foods help clean the teeth and gums.
- If your loved one has forgotten how to brush, provide easy instructions. You can brush your teeth at the same time and let the individual mimic your actions, from placing the toothpaste on the brush to brushing and rinsing. Some patients seem to like to use an electric toothbrush better than brushing on their own.
- If the handle of the toothbrush is too difficult to grip, you can purchase big-grip brushes from specialty stores, or you can wrap duct or masking tape around the handle of a regular toothbrush to make it thicker.
- Some medications cause dry mouth, which can promote tooth decay and other dental problems. Talk to your doctor about this possibility. If the offensive medication cannot be changed, make sure your loved one drinks small amounts of water throughout the day to prevent problems.
- If your loved one wears dentures and they are causing gum problems or pain, talk to the dentist about getting them adjusted. Some people with Alzheimer's disease refuse to wear their dentures because the dentures hurt, and a simple adjustment can make wearing them possible.

Wearing their dentures also will improve their ability to chew and thus digest their food better.

Falls

The tendency to fall increases with age, and people who have Alzheimer's disease are twice as likely to fracture their hip than individuals their age who do not have the disease. Because some people with Alzheimer's are confused or they become frightened or agitated, they may be more likely to stumble, fall off a chair or bed, cut themselves, or walk into furniture. If any of these accidents occur without you witnessing them, any injuries may go unnoticed if your loved one forgets or refuses to tell you. (Falls may also be related to arrhythmias; see "Cardiovascular Conditions" in this chapter.)

Preventing such injuries is your first line of defense (see the box, "How to Prevent Falls and Other Accidents"), and your second line is to be observant. If you or another caregiver helps with dressing or bathing, these are opportunities to look for any bruises, abrasions, cuts, scrapes, or other signs of injury or illness. Depending on how cooperative or communicative the patient is, you can ask, "Does anything hurt today?" or "Did you fall down this morning?" and "Can you show me where you bumped (cut, hurt, burned) yourself?"

Finally, because osteoporosis (bone loss) and risk for fractures are very high in the elderly, talk to your doctor about prevention and treatment of osteoporosis.

How to Prevent Falls and Other Accidents

If you are caring for your loved one at home, you'll need to safeguard the living and outdoor areas where he or she may frequent to help prevent falls and other accidents. Here are some guidelines:

- Remove throw rugs from living areas. Also remove welcome mats from entrance areas.
- Make sure all carpeting is securely attached to the floor. Repair any turned-up edges or wrinkles.
- Keep all telephone and electrical wires taped down or away from walking or sitting areas.
- Place no-slip strips in the bottom of the shower stall and bathtub. Safety grab bars may also be necessary in these areas.
- Use a shower chair in the bathtub or shower if your loved one has difficulty with balance or standing.
- Make sure all hallways, stairways, and other walkway areas are well lit at night.
- Use night lights to light the way to the bathroom at night. Keep a lamp or flashlight at the bedside so it can be turned on in the middle of the night as needed.
- If your loved one has a tendency to wander, you might install a bell at the top of all doors (out of reach of the individual) that lead to the outside so you will be alerted when he or she tries to leave the house. If necessary, you may need to lock such doors.
- If all the fixtures in your bathroom are the same or a similar color (e.g., a white sink, toilet, and bathtub), you can help individuals distinguish between them by applying decals to them.

- Place brightly colored tape on the edge of the bottom step of all stairways in and outside your home.
- Install handrails on all stairways.
- Have your loved one wear sturdy, flat shoes with crepe soles. Walking and athletic shoes are generally the best. Avoid heels and shoes with open toes.
- Encourage your loved one to take care when getting up from a lying position. He or she should sit up slowly, sit on the edge of the bed for a minute or two, then stand up slowly and stand still for a few seconds before walking.
- If your loved one should fall, remain calm. Look for signs of injury, such as abrasions, cuts, swelling, redness, bruises, or broken bones. If you believe there is a head injury or broken bones, call for emergency medical assistance. If your loved one does not appear to be injured, you can encourage him or her to stand unassisted.
- Keep emergency numbers (ambulance, fire, neighbors or family members who can assist in an emergency) next to the telephone and listed on your refrigerator at all times.

Weight Loss

This is a very common problem among the elderly and among Alzheimer's patients in particular. I have found that maintaining an ideal body weight is key to preventing falls, maintaining muscle strength and mobility, and for general well-being. Weight should be monitored monthly. If there is significant weight loss (more than three pounds over a month), I advocate aggressive regaining of weight through the use of supplements like Ensure as well as more traditional methods of weight gain like ice cream. It is my opinion that in these situations, the risks associated with weight loss are more serious than the risks associated with the consumption of high-calorie, high-fat, and high-protein foods for the period of time needed to regain weight.

Pressure Sores

Also known as bedsores, these painful skin conditions can develop among people who must sit or lie down for prolonged periods of time. They typically appear among people who are bedridden or wheelchair-bound, but they can be a problem for individuals who have some mobility but who stay in the same position for many hours at a time.

Bedsores begin as red, swollen areas of skin that have contact with a bed or chair, but they can quickly become open sores and infected if they are left unattended. Keep these tips in mind:

- If your loved one is confined to a bed or wheelchair most or all of the time, it's important that you check for bedsores daily. This can be done during dressing or bathing. The most common location for these sores is the buttocks.
- If your loved one is sedentary, the best way to avoid bedsores is to reposition him or her about every two hours. You may need a friend, family member, or home health aide to help you with this task. You can learn tips from a home health aide, nurse, or physical therapist on how to safely and comfortably reposition your loved one. Talk to your doctor or nurse about having someone come to your home to show you proper procedures and items that can assist you, such as foam or gel pads, pillows, padded cups

for the heels and elbows, air mattresses and egg carton mattress pads.

- Alternatively, chairs are available that can be positioned at different settings to facilitate even weight distribution and prevent sores.
- Pressure sores can also develop from wearing poorly fitted or tight clothing. Because people with Alzheimer's disease often can't communicate that something is bothering them, ill-fitting shoes, clothing, or even jewelry may cause sores to develop before they are noticed. Make sure these items are comfortable for your loved one.

THE BOTTOM LINE

People who have Alzheimer's disease typically also have other medical conditions—sometimes major diseases, oftentimes minor ailments as well—that can complicate their care and disrupt their lives and the lives of their caregivers. Thus proper attention to these health issues is critical.

If your loved one has a medical condition that is not receiving professional attention, talk to your doctor immediately. If you do not get satisfaction, ask to see a specialist, such as a geriatrician, who specializes in the diagnosis and treatment of health problems of the elderly. It is also important that you ensure your loved one has regular checkups and routine examinations for dental, vision, and hearing problems. These examinations can help anticipate and avoid health difficulties down the road.

Chapter 11

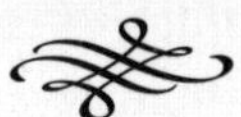

Dealing with Challenging Behaviors

The impact of Alzheimer's disease can extend far beyond the individual who has the condition. In most cases that I see in my practice, Alzheimer's disease is a family concern: a spouse, son, daughter, grandchild, or other family member—or a close friend—takes on the role of caregiver. In fact, more than half of the people in the United States who have Alzheimer's disease are cared for by family and/or friends at home.

In one way this is a beautiful thing: there is a profound closeness, warmth, and love that can permeate the experience of living with and caring for someone who has Alzheimer's disease. Families and friends can learn to appreciate the good times of the past and create new ones for the present and future.

Caregiving also has its challenges. Generally, caregivers—the majority of whom are women—are forced to learn as they go along, discovering new things about the disease and its impact on their loved one—and themselves—one day at a time.

The toll these new responsibilities can take on people who are often working full-time, managing their own homes and families, or who may be elderly or frail themselves, can be staggering. Often they devote so much of their time and energy to the patient that they neglect themselves, physically, emotionally, and spiritually. Thus caregivers need and deserve all the support and guidance they can get.

In this chapter I share some of the advice and guidelines I offer the families and friends of people who have Alzheimer's. Specifically, we will look at some of the challenging behaviors that are present in some patients with Alzheimer's disease and how to deal with them. Practicing effective coping strategies can help make your loved one's life as meaningful and rewarding as possible, and can improve your quality of life and your relationship with the person who has Alzheimer's disease. No one can guarantee the success of any of the guidance offered here; some tips may work one day and not the next; they may work with your mother but not your friend's father. That's just the unpredictable nature of the disease. But if you are armed with basic management skills, you are much more likely to be successful most of the time.

I believe the Alzheimer's Association is the best organization of its kind for helping, educating, and providing multifaceted support for caregivers. The association has chapters in most areas of the United States where caregiver support groups are run as a forum for education but also as a place to vent and to be with individuals who are in a similar situation. It is also the biggest funder of research outside of the government, with the goal of finding ways to deal more effectively with this illness. A nonprofit organization staffed by both employees and volunteers, the association is funded by donations from private individuals. I encourage people to utilize the services of this organization and to support its efforts.

A RANDOM ACT OF UNKINDNESS

One characteristic of Alzheimer's disease is that as it progresses, different parts of the brain are affected in an apparently random way. The unpredictable nature of cell damage in the brain results in behaviors that don't make sense to us or to the person who has Alzheimer's disease. This seemingly arbitrary destruction of brain cells can also cause various behavioral changes. It is important to note that many patients with Alzheimer's disease may never experience these changes and certainly not in the early stages. Most patients may experience some of the symptoms some of the time especially in the advanced stages of Alzheimer's.

A Return to Childhood

I believe there is something kind about Alzheimer's disease in that it brings people back to their childhood. This may sound like an odd statement to make; however, if people had a good or decent childhood, then "going back" to that time can be a pleasant, even sweet experience. When you think about what it means to be a child—having parents take care of you, having your needs provided for, having friends and summer vacations—then you can see how returning to those times in one's mind can be an enjoyable thing.

As people make that mental trip back in time toward childhood, they pass through other memories. Habits and behaviors individuals had engaged in years ago may return, such as preparing to go to work in the morning or taking up smoking even though they may have quit decades ago. Some people who speak English as a second language may revert back to speaking their native language, although this is very uncommon. These behaviors can be viewed as simply being part of the backward journey people with Alzheimer's disease may make, a permanent stroll down memory lane, if you will.

At a biological level, this return to childhood can be simplistically viewed as reaching deep into the brain, where long-term memories are stored. As we discussed earlier in the book, the parts of the brain that store short-term memory are generally damaged before those that harbor very long-term (childhood) memories. As short-term memory fades, these very long-term stored memories come to the surface, so to speak.

Apraxia

One of my major goals when talking with caregivers is to educate them about apraxia—the loss of ability to perform regular, everyday tasks. Something seemingly as simple as brushing one's teeth, putting on a pair of pants, or using a spoon can become difficult to some persons with Alzheimer's disease. For example: A person with apraxia will begin to perform a task, say, brush his teeth. He picks up the toothbrush, as he has done every day for much of his life. He reaches for the toothpaste and suddenly stops. He stares at the tube of toothpaste, then brings it to his mouth and begins to move it across his teeth. Or he may simply put down the toothbrush and the toothpaste and walk away without completing the task.

Apraxia may be present one day and not the next, one minute and not the next. It is important for caregivers to be aware of this. Too often, because of this variability and the seeming simplicity of the task, exhausted and frustrated caregivers will say, "He is doing it on purpose! I know he knows how to brush his teeth" (or use a fork, brush his hair, and so on). However, the individual is *not* choosing to be difficult.

People who have apraxia can't complete a task because the signals created in the brain (specifically, in the cerebral cortex and, on occasion, subcortical structures) break down, the person becomes distracted, and the task is not completed. Thus when your mother tries to butter her bread with a fork, your father picks up the telephone and begins to talk without dialing anyone, your grandmother has trouble with figuring out how to put on her jacket, or your dear friend has trouble opening a door, apraxia is probably at work.

The best thing you can do in situations like these is, first, stay calm and remember that your loved one isn't being defiant or intentionally difficult. Then, gently help the individual complete the task he or she has started. Do not make negative comments or criticize the attempt that was made. Once the task is complete, let your loved one continue on with his or her day.

When Brenda noticed that her father had picked up a comb, stopped, and then stared at it without knowing what to do, she patted him gently on the back. "Yes, your hair does need to be combed, Dad," she said as she took his hand that held the comb. She then helped him draw the comb through his hair several times until he could do it on his own. "Looks great, Dad. Now, would you like some lunch?"

Hemi-Neglect

Some patients with Alzheimer's disease experience what is called a "hemi-neglect," a reduced ability or an inability to hear, understand, see, or otherwise interact with their environment on one side of their body. In almost all cases, the neglect occurs on the left side of the body, corresponding to right-side brain (parietal lobe) damage. For reasons related to brain specialization, left-sided brain damage does not cause neglect of the right side of the body!

Hemi-neglect, unless identified and explained to patients and families, can be frustrating for all concerned, with significant caregiving repercussions. I myself came upon its implications accidentally when, in the process of cognitive rehabilitation, I found that some patients will do much better when I sit on their right rather than on their left. The impact of hemi-neglect on caregiving is rarely discussed in books or articles on Alzheimer's disease. Yet it can be a frustrating and confusing thing for caregivers unless they understand what is happening.

Therefore, I tell caregivers about this phenomenon and instruct them to take notice if their loved one is having difficulty with his or her left side. Sometimes neglect first becomes noticeable when patients don't respond when people talk to them on their left side. Some individuals completely ignore anything that appears on the left pages in a book or magazine or food on the left side of their plate. People with Alzheimer's may become startled when someone approaches them on their left side.

If your loved one seems to have hemi-neglect, there are some adjustments you and others who are in the company of the person who has Alzheimer's disease can make to circumvent it. These include:

- Approaching individuals on their right side
- Speaking to individuals from the right side
- Walking with them on their right side
- Placing items on their right side (e.g., food on the table, clothing on the bed, comb and brush on the vanity)
- Reminding family members, other caregivers, and anyone else who interacts with the patient to approach from the right side

CHALLENGING BEHAVIORS

"Why does my husband act happy and calm one minute and then start screaming at me the next?"

"My mother turned around and hit her neighbor today for

no reason at all. When I asked her why she did it, she didn't even know what I was talking about."

"Yesterday my brother kept yelling that someone had stolen his watch and his clothes. When we showed him his watch and clothes, he still kept insisting someone had stolen them, that these weren't his things."

"I discovered that my father was hiding food all around the house. I found sandwiches and cookies under his bed, rotting bananas in the linen closet under a pile of towels."

"My wife seems to have lost all her inhibitions. Whenever she needs to go to the bathroom, she tries to unzip her pants, even if we are standing in a restaurant."

"Sometimes in the morning, my mother gets dressed and goes out to the car as if she's going to drive to her old job at the local high school. She's been retired for fifteen years."

These are just a few examples of the types of challenging behaviors people with Alzheimer's disease may engage in. The following discussion is not meant to frighten you, and it by no means represents behaviors that are guaranteed to happen to everyone who has Alzheimer's disease. Progression of the disease can vary dramatically from person to person. Every individual is different, and how each person interacts with his or her environment, medications, and other therapies all have an effect on behavior.

Getting a Grip on Difficult Behaviors

"When my husband begins to shout and get bossy with me," says Verna, a seventy-five-year-old retired seamstress whose eighty-year-old husband, Charles, often tests her patience, "I grit my teeth and say to myself, 'Time to make lemonade out of lemons.' A sense of humor and a willingness to try some creative ways to manage difficult behaviors—that's what works for me." In the following sections we offer some suggestions on how to deal with specific types of difficult behaviors, and we add a section that discusses general coping strategies.

One suggestion many caregivers find helpful is to keep a notebook in which to jot down information about specific behaviors. This can help you "get a grip" on the situation. You should take notes on:

- What seems to precipitate certain behaviors
- How the person acts—the movements, gestures, and other actions; whether they are repetitive or random
- What he or she may say
- Time of day the behavior occurs
- Who was present
- Environment (location of the behavior, such as the store, home, park, church)
- What seems to help end the behavior

Keeping a written account of such information can be very helpful in noticing any trends and can provide you with effective hints on how to modify disruptive behaviors.

Anger, Aggression, and Defiance: Pick Your Battles

Being a caregiver is a challenging role, and one thing I always stress to family and friends who are in this position is to pick their battles and set their priorities. That's the advice I gave Harold, whose fifty-two-year-old wife, Janice, became aggressive two years after she was diagnosed with early-onset Alzheimer's disease. Harold called me one morning and said that Janice had been refusing to eat her meals, and when he tried to force her, she hit him. He was terrified that she would go hungry and get sick, and he didn't know what to do.

I assured him that as Janice had not lost any weight, missing a few meals would not place her in any medical danger, and that he should stop forcing her to eat. Instead, he should get some foods that she likes and leave them where she could easily get them—on the kitchen counter or in plain view in the refrigerator. She would eat when she was hungry. At mealtimes, I suggested he place a small amount in front of her, and if she ate it, fine; if not, he was to put the platter in the refrigerator for later.

This approach worked for Janice: Harold had far fewer "food fights" on his hands, Janice maintained a relatively nutritious diet, and the stress level for both husband and wife is much lower than it was.

When people who have Alzheimer's disease become angry, they may sometimes act out by hitting, throwing objects, shouting, slamming things, or making accusations. The most effective way to defuse such situations is to act calmly. If you reply with anger, it will only fuel the behavior that is directed at you. The next step is to remove the fuel. In Harold and Janice's case, the "fuel" was Harold's pressure to make his wife eat. Once he stopped trying to force her, she ate on her own. Also, keep notes on each occasion, as it may help you identify different triggers or ways to prevent or defuse future episodes.

I talk with many caregivers who ask me why their loved ones are angry at them. "There doesn't seem to be any reason," they say. "I'm just trying to help them."

People with Alzheimer's disease who become angry often act out because they are actually frightened, frustrated, or confused. Their sense of reality is threatened or they don't understand what they are seeing or hearing. Thus what a caregiver sees and understands as something perfectly normal is seen and interpreted by the person with Alzheimer's in a very different, and sometimes threatening or frightening way.

Wandering

Wandering is often called the most frustrating problem behavior associated with Alzheimer's disease, because not only can it place the individual in physical danger, it can also make it impossible for adult day care centers to care for or even admit individuals who engage in it. It is also stressful for caregivers, whose lives and sleep are often disrupted by wandering behavior, and who worry about the safety of their loved one.

Fortunately, there are some effective ways to control wandering behavior. The secret is to understand *why* the person is wandering. Common reasons include:

- Going "home," a symbolic place where one is free from cares or worries, rather than a geographic place. This is the most common reason for wandering.
- Side effect of medication
- Restlessness
- Agitation
- Anxiety
- Fear, caused by an inability to interpret sounds and images around the person
- Desire to perform some task or obligation from their past, such as going to work, picking up a child at school, or running errands
- Boredom
- Need for exercise
- Recent change in living arrangements, e.g., moving to a new city, into a nursing home, or into the home of a family member
- Pain, discomfort, or illness that he/she can't communicate
- Searching for things he/she has lost or can't find

Discovering why your loved one is wandering may take some detective work, and judicious use of your notebook is important here. Beatrice kept careful notes for several days before she uncovered the cause of her husband Tom's wandering behavior.

"At first I thought he wandered because he's always liked to walk," says Beatrice. "So I wasn't even going to bother keeping notes. I started taking a long walk with him every afternoon, but that didn't end his wandering. In fact, he seemed even more restless. I began to write down what was going on."

That's when Beatrice noticed that during their walks, Tom would stop and stare at the cars going by or those in parking lots. At first Beatrice didn't think this was important, but then she realized that her husband was fixated on red cars. When he saw one he'd mumble to himself, but Beatrice never understood what he was saying.

"Our daughter, Candice, had a red car," says Beatrice. "She was killed fifty years ago in an automobile accident. I listened carefully to what Tom was saying whenever he saw a red car, and I realized it was 'Candy' over and over. I assumed his wandering was related to trying to find our daughter."

Although Beatrice couldn't bring her daughter back, she tried something else. "Some people might think what I did was strange, but it worked. I gathered together pictures of our daughter and arranged them in one corner of our study—framed pictures and photo albums. Then I got a model of a red car and put posters of red cars on the walls. Tom rarely wanders anymore. Sometimes we sit together and look at pictures of our daughter, and that seems to help him a great deal."

Once you believe you've found the cause of the wandering behavior, you can try different tactics to end it, gently but firmly. See "The Bottom Line" at the end of this chapter for general approaches. In Tom's case, Beatrice redirected his reason for wandering. Some people find that reducing the amount of stress in their loved one's environment eliminates the agitation and wandering. Each person is different, and so a trial-and-error approach may be necessary until an effective method is found.

Some caregivers get a great deal of satisfaction from doing the type of "detective work" that Beatrice used to uncover her husband's reason for wandering. For some, being able to "get inside the head" of their loved one helps them better understand why the individual is acting out and also gives them clues, as it did for Beatrice, as to how they can better manage challenging behaviors. As Beatrice explains, "Once I found out why Tom was acting in what seemed to be a bizarre way, it didn't seem so strange anymore. I could understand why he was acting the way he was. The experience of discovering the reason for his strange behavior has actually made us closer. I feel less impatient, and I think Tom feels that some of the stress has been lifted."

Regardless of the reasons for wandering, there are some general guidelines I encourage caregivers to follow, both for their safety and that of their loved one.

- I encourage everyone to enroll their loved one in the Safe Return Program offered by the Alzheimer's Association. This is a nationwide, federally funded program that provides identifying labels, a national photo and information database, 24-hour toll-free emergency hotline, and wandering behavior education and training for caregivers. See the Appendix.
- Individuals who choose not to enroll in the Safe Return Program should take other measures to ensure the safety of their loved one, including making sure people with Alzheimer's disease have some form of identification on them at all times. The best type is something they can't lose or throw away. Identifying labels (name, address, and

phone) sewn into their clothing are effective. A Medic-Alert bracelet is another alternative. Often, patients who refuse to wear a bracelet (especially men) will agree to a dog tag. A simple piece of silver or gold jewelry with the patient's name and a telephone number engraved on it may be an acceptable, dignified alternative for the patient.

- Always keep a recent picture of your loved one available should he/she wander away and you need to call the police for help.
- Childproof doorknobs and window safety latches, available at hardware stores, may be necessary for escape routes that may lead to potential danger. These can be operated quickly in case of fire or other emergency by people who are not confused.
- Medication to prevent wandering should be used quickly and effectively when behavioral methods fail.
- If your loved one gets lost and is returned to you, don't scold or yell. People with Alzheimer's disease don't get lost on purpose, and they are often very frightened by the entire event. As the caregiver, you need to reassure your loved one and get both of you back to a normal routine as quickly as possible.

Hoarding, Hiding, and Losing Things

Cookies in the laundry basket. Car keys in potted plants. A collection of empty cans under the bed. Some persons with Alzheimer's disease frequently will hide, lose, or hoard everyday objects, which can be especially frustrating for you and other family members. "My wife keeps hiding my socks," says William, who cares for his eighty-one-year-old wife, Yolanda. "Why does she do that?"

William has asked a question that is the same or similar to

others caregivers everywhere ask their loved ones: "Why did you do that?" or "Where did you put the ____?" or "Why are you collecting _____?" My advice to you is, don't expect an answer. When William asks Yolanda why she is hiding and hoarding his socks, she can't tell him verbally. Yet in a way she *is* telling him. Yolanda isn't hoarding socks because she likes socks but because they represent something special to her, and in this case that "something" is her husband.

Some people with Alzheimer's disease hoard objects that remind them of something pleasant, familiar, or safe, such as stuffed animals or certain pieces of clothing. One woman, Lorraine, hoarded chocolate chip cookies; she didn't eat them, she just collected them in her closet. Why? Because that's what her grandmother used to bake for her when she was a child. Once her caregiver, Gerry, understood why Lorraine collected the cookies (which were attracting ants in the closet), she got Lorraine an airtight plastic container into which she could continue to collect and place the cookies in the closet, safe from ants.

Please remember, there is no rational reason for hiding and hoarding behaviors. But there are ways you can, like Gerry, make the best of them without making a big deal out of them, which will only upset your loved one. For example, Connie's husband, Ron, kept taking the coffee cups out of the kitchen cabinet and putting them in the hall closet. Her solution: she put a childproof doorknob on the hall closet door so Ron couldn't open it. After discovering he couldn't put the cups into the hall closet, he put them into the bedroom closet. She then put childproof knobs on all the closet doors in the house. When Ron found he couldn't hide the cups in the closets, he stopped taking the cups out of the kitchen cabinet.

Here are a few helpful tips:

- As a backup measure, you should always keep spares of important items, such as car and house keys, eyeglasses, dentures, and hearing aid batteries. Store these items in a locked box or other secure place.
- Reduce the number of places your loved one can hide items by locking (or using childproof doorknobs) on some closets and rooms. Childproof latches can be used on cabinets and drawers.
- Don't keep much cash around the house.
- Safely secure in a locked box or room or remove altogether valuable items such as jewelry, coins, or collectibles.
- Make it a habit to check wastepaper baskets and trash cans before you dispose of their contents.
- Periodically check under mattresses, sofa and chair cushions, and in laundry baskets for hidden items.

Sexually Inappropriate Behavior

It is rare for true sexual acting out to occur among people who have Alzheimer's disease. More commonly, behavior that can be construed as sexually inappropriate but in fact is not related to sex can occur. For instance, a woman may unbutton her blouse if hot, or if she feels it is uncomfortable, or if she thinks it is time to change or take a shower or go to bed. A man may unzip his pants in public because he needs to go to the bathroom. Redirection and reassurance is needed, as is discerning the true needs of the individual.

Sometimes changing the person's clothing discourages inappropriate behaviors. Men can wear pants that pull on instead of those with a zipper, and women might avoid tops that have buttons down the front. Having the patient dress appropriately for weather or environmental conditions can also help. If you know that your aunt tends to feel warm even when a room doesn't feel warm to you, you might have her wear a short-sleeved top but bring along a sweater just in case she needs it later.

Repetitive Actions or Speech

"If he asks me that question one more time, I'm going to scream." I've heard this statement, or variations thereof, many times, and the frustration in the people's voices is obvious and understandable. Patients will often ask, "Where are you going?" or "When will you come back?" or "Why can't I go with you?" or similar questions. One thing that's common among these types of questions is that they voice fear. Once you understand that your loved one repeats the same phrase or question out of anxiety or fear, you are more likely to be empathetic rather than frustrated. When you are more calm and less frustrated, those feelings can be felt by the person who has Alzheimer's disease, and it can help reduce their frustrations as well.

Sometimes people with Alzheimer's disease keep repeating certain behaviors or activities, such as constantly folding clothes, pacing back and forth, or tapping their fingers on a table. If your loved one is doing repetitive behaviors, your task is twofold: stay calm, and break the cycle, in that order. If you become upset and chastise your loved one, he or she may become more agitated, and you will not achieve your goal. Instead, try gentle diversion. Isadore's aunt, Clara, repeatedly asked, "When are we going to Dallas?" sometimes twenty or thirty times a day. Isadore soon learned that saying, "We can't go to Dallas" or "We'll go tomorrow," or just ignoring her only made her aunt agitated and caused her to shout the question more and more.

Instead, Isadore switched to an "answer a question with a question" approach. "Now when my aunt asks the question, I ask her, 'What would you like to do in Dallas?' or 'What's your favorite place in Dallas?' and she answers me," says Isadore. "She seems to enjoy answering the questions, she forgets the question she asked me, and we avoid arguments and confrontations." Unfortunately, this method does not always work.

People who engage in repetitive actions can also be distracted with a new activity, but it should be done in a nonthreatening, nonpressured way. You might suggest that he or she "help" you with a chore, like folding clothes. It's okay if the individual keeps refolding the same clothes again and again, because the repetitive action often helps them achieve a sense of calm, control, and order in a world that has become chaotic and incomprehensible to them. Stacking coins or rearranging books on a shelf may also help.

Paranoia, False Ideas, and Suspicions

Marie called the police and told them that her neighbor was stealing the silverware from her house. Martin kept telling everyone in the family that his wife of fifty years, Sophia, was cheating on him with the TV repairman. When Doris is in a room with people, she insists everyone is talking about her.

On occasion, some people with Alzheimer's disease may become overly suspicious or even paranoid. They may insist upon seemingly unreasonable ideas, like Lydia, who sits on the porch every morning and waits for her mother, who has been dead for more than twenty years. Such behaviors can be very upsetting to caregivers and family members, because they equate them with "craziness" or "losing one's mind." However, these beliefs are actually an attempt by the brain to deal with a loss—the death of a parent or spouse, moving away from a home someone lived in for decades, a failure to remember names and faces, or even the ability to control one's own life.

This mechanism of defense occurs in all of us. For example, when we cannot find items frequently, we may blame it on someone or something (the new housekeeper, the new roommate, lack of sleep). Alternatively, if we cannot find a parked car in a parking lot and we are sure we parked it there, we may suspect it is stolen or that it was towed, rather than faulting ourselves and our minds for misremembering where we parked the car.

Various tactics can help you cope with suspicious and paranoid behaviors. **Your responses should always be nonconfrontational.** This can take some practice, as it is natural to defend yourself when someone is attacking you verbally or making false accusations. Do not tell your loved one he or she is wrong or lying. If your mother insists that someone has stolen all her jewelry, don't say, "No one stole it. I've told you that a hundred times." Instead, you can remind her that she had her valuables placed in a safe deposit box and then show her the key. Then gently change the subject.

Because suspicions, false ideas, and paranoia are how individuals express confusion and fear, your response might address those feelings. A husband who unjustly believes that his spouse is being unfaithful may need some reassurance that his wife still loves him, which can be as simple as sitting with him and holding his hand or giving him hugs throughout the day and telling him how special he is to her. Finally, medications are very effective in treating these symptoms.

Clinging

Sometimes spouses and family members tell me how their loved ones follow them around the house and make it impossible to be alone or get away without causing a scene. Heidi, a lovely seventy-three-year-old retired teacher, complained how her husband, Eric, wouldn't let her out of his sight. "He even tries to follow me into the bathroom. I feel guilty locking him out, and then I worry because he sits and cries outside the door. He wants to go everywhere with me. He even resents it when someone comes over to visit. He constantly interrupts our conversation and must be the center of attention."

Individuals who cling to their caregivers are acting out their fear. Time has little meaning to them, so if you say, "I'll be right back," they don't know what that means, and they become frightened. If you disappear from their sight, they don't understand that you'll come back.

Several tactics may be helpful. The clinging is the result of anxiety and fear, not insecurity. Offering reassurances throughout the day that they are loved and valued may be beneficial. Offer distractions that may hold their interest, such as drawing or painting or music (art can be an effective distraction; see chapter 9). Writing down on a piece of paper exactly what time you will be back and where you are going is helpful for some patients. The paper can be posted on the refrigerator or kept next to the person on a table or nightstand for reassurance.

Clinging behavior can be very stressful for caregivers. If you have a clinging loved one, it's important that you get some relief and time away. Some hints are offered in chapter 12.

THE BOTTOM LINE

Some people who have Alzheimer's disease may find any changes in routine to be overwhelming, confusing, and chaotic. When a person's brain isn't able to process information the way it once did, is it any wonder he or she would be angry or afraid, and thus act out those feelings? In this chapter we looked at some specific types of challenging behaviors and ways to deal with them. But how you handle these behaviors—and others we didn't discuss—can be broken down into seven general areas. I believe you'll find that if you adopt one or more of these guidelines when difficult behaviors or emotions arise, you'll often be rewarded with promising results.

Create a Routine

One of the primary characteristics of Alzheimer's disease is the loss of control—of one's thoughts, emotions, and actions. One way to help restore a sense of control for your loved one is to establish and follow some routines or rituals on a daily and weekly basis. Routines give patients something they can rely on and about which they can feel secure and safe. Include activities that are enjoyable, such as taking a walk every night before dinner, watching a favorite television show, tending the garden after breakfast, going to the library every Monday, or attending religious services.

Distract, Redirect

Sometimes you can distract or redirect a person's attention from an unacceptable activity toward something positive or constructive. Individuals who are agitated, restless, or wandering may respond if you redirect their energies into an activity such as raking leaves, sweeping the patio, or folding the laundry. Introduce a creative activity, such as painting with watercolors, drawing with charcoal, or planting flower seeds (see chapter 9, "Stimulating the Senses").

Offer Reassurance

Everyone has the need to feel loved and secure, and these needs are especially important to people for whom these positive feelings are slipping away. Reassurance can be offered in many forms, from being attentive when the person with Alzheimer's is talking to offering hugs or pats on the hand or shoulder throughout the day. Simple, sincere phrases such as "You're special to me," "We're glad you're part of the family," or "We love you, Mom" even once a day can mean a lot to people who feel alone and afraid.

Reduce Stress

Today's fast-paced, chaotic lifestyle is often overwhelming for many of us, so imagine what it feels like to those with cognitive impairment. Overstimulation from their surroundings, including noisy public places (e.g., restaurants, department stores, ball games, concerts, fairs), a chaotic home environment (playing radios, stereos, and televisions simultaneously), or even taking your loved one along on a series of errands may provide too many sensory signals for them to process without feeling frightened, confused, or agitated.

Note the circumstances under which the person with Alzheimer's displays these behaviors and feelings; or, conversely, observe how he or she behaves when in such situations. Then take steps to reduce the stressors. For example, instead of going to a restaurant, you could pack a picnic and eat in the park, or choose a quiet restaurant and go at off hours. At home, if the television or radio bothers the patient, keep the volume down as low as possible, use earphones, or close the doors in rooms to keep the noise to a minimum. Naturally, his or her response to stressors may change as the disease progresses, so you will need to be alert to changes in response.

Keep It Simple

Tasks that were once simple to do or directions that were once easy to follow can become complex mysteries to people who have Alzheimer's disease. Monica's father, who was diagnosed with Alzheimer's five years ago, used to become increasingly frustrated when his daughter tried to tell him how to get dressed.

"I'd tell him to put on his pants, and he'd just stare at me, or sometimes he'd become agitated and wave his arms and yell. Then I'd try to help him, and he'd cry or try to hit me. I dreaded every confrontation." Then someone in Monica's support group told her to simplify her message. "Now I say, 'Dad, sit on the bed. Now put your left leg into the pant leg. Now put your right leg into the other pant leg. Now stand up.' I do this every time, and surprisingly, his getting dressed takes less time than it used to when we were battling all the time."

Keeping it simple is not the same as being condescending. It is my opinion that nothing is more of a tragedy than for someone with an illness like Alzheimer's disease to feel patronized. To an individual threatened with loss of dignity, this is often terrible. Always treat your loved one as an adult; he or she just needs to hear directions in smaller, more manageable segments. Some caregivers have remarked that having to give directions in this manner has made them appreciate how complicated some of our routine, everyday tasks really are.

"I no longer get shoes for my father that need to be tied," says Robert. "When I realized how difficult it was to explain to my father how to tie a shoe, I ran out and bought him loafers and shoes with Velcro. We take so many things for granted, like tying our shoes or preparing a bowl of cereal. I'm appreciating my dad and everything he's still able to do so much more now."

Safety

Childproof latches can be put on drawers and cabinets, and childproof doorknobs are also available. Safety locks can also be placed on the oven and stove (see the Appendix), or you may choose to remove knobs from these appliances or even pull the plug or throw the circuit breakers when they are not in use.

Shift Perspective

Sometimes, your attempts to redirect, distract, simplify, console, or create routines don't work, especially as individuals enter the latter stage of the disease. That's when you may need to shift your perspective—look at the glass as being half full instead of half empty, so to speak—when dealing with challenging behaviors and emotional outbursts from your loved one. Although it is helpful to be ever mindful that the disease is causing the difficult behaviors, it is, as one caregiver said, "one thing to *know intellectually* why my husband does the things he does, but quite another to *accept them emotionally.*"

To shift your perspective, focus on what you know about the disease or, better yet, what you can learn that can help your loved one and you live day to day, rather than focus on all the things you don't understand. When you take active steps to learn and understand—when you read this book and follow the exercises and suggestions, attend support groups, ask for help from family and friends, work closely with medical professionals—you take some control of the situation rather than being controlled by it.

Like the progression of any chronic disease, Alzheimer's presents changes over time: in behavior, moods, physical abilities, and cognitive functioning. As a caregiver, shifting your perspective as the disease unfolds can be challenging, and how to handle those challenges is the topic of the next chapter, in which we talk about how to take care of *you.*

Medications

Several medications are effective and safe in treating these behaviors. When behavioral treatments are not effective, please talk to your physician about using an appropriate medication.

Chapter 12

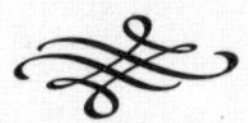

Coming to the Aid of Caregivers

I believe caring for a person who has Alzheimer's disease is one of the most challenging, important, and rewarding jobs on earth. Every day, I have the privilege of speaking and working with spouses, partners, sons, daughters, other family members, and friends who care for loved ones, and I share with them their stories and concerns. While the health and welfare of the patients is certainly important, so too is the physical, emotional, and spiritual well-being of their caregivers.

So this chapter is just for you, a time to ask you, "How's it going? What are your concerns? What do you need for you to cope or feel better?" We will talk about how you can care for yourself: where to look for help, ways to prevent physical and emotional stress, and how to deal with feelings of guilt, remorse, fear, anxiety, and frustration. Included in our discussion are two topics many caregivers find hard to talk about: maintaining sexual relations with their partner, and physical aggression by caregivers against their loved ones. Some caregivers have become my heroes and heroines, people who give me inspiration to continue on and to look up to.

HIRING HELP

What characteristics should you look for when hiring someone to care for your loved one? That was the question facing Glenda, whose father had been diagnosed with Alzheimer's disease three years ago.

Glenda called me on the phone and said she had a dilemma. Her ninety-two-year-old father, Marvin, lived alone in his own apartment, and she lived more than a hundred miles away. Glenda works full-time, but she visits her father once a week and calls him several times a day to remind him to take his medications. When Glenda discovered that Marvin was not following her instructions, she decided to hire a full-time, certified home health aide to stay with her father to monitor his prescriptions and to help ensure his safety.

Marvin, who had enjoyed privacy and independence before the aide moved in, was now sharing his home with a stranger with whom he had nothing in common. On the third day of the aide's assignment, Marvin hit her when she tried to give him his medication.

Now, says Glenda, the aide has quit and she doesn't know what to do. Another family member suggested hiring a young man named Jeremy, who enjoys working with the elderly but who is not a certified health aide. Jeremy is willing to take Marvin to watch tennis tournaments (a game Marvin had once played passionately), to the theater, and for walks in the park. Marvin has met Jeremy and seems to like him. "But he's not a certified caregiver," Glenda said. "Should I hire him anyway?"

I believe the essential qualifications of a caregiver are patience, compassion, integrity, and common sense. If an individual has all these characteristics and the patient has a rapport with the person, then it doesn't matter whether the individual is certified. What matters is the safety, well-being, and quality of life of your loved one. Naturally, if specialized medical attention is required, you will need someone to handle that portion of care.

Ideally, these same qualities will be present in whoever you find to help you care for your loved one—be it a family member, friend, home health aide, or a volunteer who provides respite for you once or twice a week. Resources for finding help are listed in the Appendix.

GETTING HELP FOR YOU

It's not unusual to hear about caregivers who work so hard and diligently at helping their loved one that they become emotionally and physically ill themselves. Many caregivers are older and/or have medical conditions, full-time jobs, or families that place additional stress on an already tense situation. **That's why it's critical for anyone who has assumed caregiving responsibilities to learn how to take care of their physical, emotional, and spiritual needs.** After all, you won't be able to help your loved one if you yourself are ill.

Respite

The most important thing caregivers can do for themselves is schedule regular respite—at least once a week, and ideally more frequently. Respite should include time away from the caregiving environment and doing something that you enjoy, relieves your stress, and/or provides you comfort. Take a walk, visit friends, go shopping, see a movie, get a massage. If possible, establish a regular respite time each week so you'll have that to look forward to. Marion, whose sixty-nine-year-old husband, Franklin, has been living with Alzheimer's for four years, goes to a senior center every Tuesday and Friday morning for a line dance class.

"I so look forward to those few hours each week," says Marion. "I used to feel guilty about taking time away from Franklin, but I know I'm much better able to deal with him if I get away for a while. I found a wonderful volunteer from a local service organization who comes to stay with my husband. When I get home from dancing I feel refreshed. Even if class is canceled for some reason, I still go out for those two hours twice a week—to a movie, shopping, or to the park. It's my time."

Respite for you can also mean arranging for your loved one to attend adult day care one or more times a week. Banish the thought that this is a selfish act: many caregivers find that their loved ones thoroughly enjoy the opportunity to socialize and participate in activities. Many day care centers offer a variety of activities that are not available to patients in their homes. Naturally, not every person who has Alzheimer's disease enjoys going to adult day care, but it is an option I suggest caregivers explore. (See the box "How to Choose Adult Day Care.")

Alzheimer's day care facilities vary in the services they offer, but basic care includes recreational activities supervised by trained professionals (e.g., music, art appreciation, crafts, gardening, dancing) and meals. Some provide transportation, field trips, and assistance with personal care such as bathing.

How to Choose Adult Day Care

- Begin to investigate adult day care facilities before you need one. It can take a while to evaluate the ones in your area, and some may have a waiting list.
- Begin your search by asking for recommendations from

your doctor, hospital, or a local or state-run aging council or department of aging (look in the telephone book). You can also contact the National Council on the Aging (202-479-1200; www.ncoa.org) or the Eldercare Locator (800-677-1116; www.eldercare.gov) for names of centers in your area.

- Visit the facility several times and at different times of the day.
- Ask to see the center's activities schedule and meal plans.
- Attend some of the activity sessions and sit in on several meals. Observe how the staff interact with the participants. Are they patient? Do they speak kindly and calmly? Do they attend to their questions and needs in a reasonable amount of time? Do the participants seem to like and enjoy the staff?
- Does the facility have the types of activities your loved one enjoys? If time with animals is very important to your loved one, for example, look for a place that offers pet therapy.
- Talk to other caregivers who have loved ones attending the facility. Ask how long they've been familiar with the center, if there have been any complaints (and if so, how they were handled), and their overall satisfaction with the facility and staff.
- Talk with staff members about concerns or questions and see if you are comfortable with their attitude and responses.
- Contact your ombudsman office (an ombudsman is a government official who handles consumer complaints) to see if there have been any complaints filed against the facility. You can find a phone number in the government pages of your phone book.

Support Groups

"I thought going to an Alzheimer's support group was going to be depressing, but I was wrong," says Nancy, who cares for her eighty-four-year-old mother at home. "We cry, we share, we even laugh, and it's all okay, because we're all in the same boat. I know this sounds strange, but when I leave a meeting, I feel uplifted, validated, understood, less helpless. I've made friends there, and we can call each other in between meetings and support each other. It's wonderful."

Nancy's sentiments are not unusual among people who attend Alzheimer's support groups. Groups are free of charge and offer a forum for people to discuss issues ranging from how to handle challenging behaviors to where to find competent adult day care or eldercare assistance. Mostly they are an opportunity for individuals to share their thoughts, frustrations, and ideas. Caregiving tips are exchanged like recipes; emotions are expressed and received with understanding. For many caregivers, such groups are their sole support outside the help they receive from medical professionals.

Most cities have a support group, typically run by the Alzheimer's Association or by hospitals, clinics, or social service agencies (see the Appendix for contact information). The Alzheimer's Association is a wonderful, not-for-profit organization that has superb services and volunteer opportunities.

If there are no groups in your area or you are unable to attend one, there are opportunities for you to get support and share information on the Internet. If you have access to the Internet, you will find various chat rooms and e-mail support groups that are dedicated to caregivers of people who have Alzheimer's disease and other forms of dementia. Many of these chat rooms and groups are run by medical professionals and/or social service organizations (see the Appendix for a list). These Internet services can be very helpful if you have limited or no access to other support in your community, although some people find they enjoy attending support groups as well as interacting on the Internet. Chat rooms and e-mail support groups allow you to contact others at any time of the day or night, at times it may not be appropriate to call someone on the telephone. Sometimes just writing an e-mail to someone and getting something off your chest is a relief.

Beware, however, of information you receive over the Internet, as it may not always be reliable. In some cases people may, either intentionally or unintentionally, give out false or even harmful information. You should check with a medical professional before following any advice someone gives you in a chat room or e-mail.

CAREGIVER AGGRESSION: HITTING BACK

Sometimes, the challenges of caring for someone with Alzheimer's disease can cause caregivers to slap, shake, shove, or scream at their loved ones. They don't mean to do it. They certainly don't plan to do it. But it happens: anger and frustration boil over and individuals lose control and their temper. They strike back at the patient, and then they have an overwhelming feeling of guilt and remorse. But they are also worried that they will do it again.

Caregiver aggression is common, yet most people, including caregivers as well as physicians, don't like to talk about it. I believe this is a grave mistake, because such aggression is simply an indication that the overburdened person needs help, and the sooner the better. This is best for both the caregivers and the patient.

Arnold and Evelyn are a good example of what happens with caregiver aggression. Arnold, an eighty-seven-year-old retired businessman, has been the primary caregiver for his wife, Evelyn, since she was diagnosed with Alzheimer's disease five years ago. Arnold dutifully brings in his eighty-two-year-old wife once a week for cognitive therapy, which she has been pursuing aggressively for more than a year. Both Arnold and Evelyn and I believe that her hard work is paying off, as her memory remains good and she continues to enjoy reading, visiting friends, and walking the dog.

Delightful as Evelyn can be, she also has many challenging behaviors. One evening, after she had been loudly repeating the same sentence over and over again for more than an hour, Arnold screamed at her to shut up. She responded by shouting even louder, at which point Arnold slapped her face. Evelyn immediately began to cry, and Arnold was filled with remorse and horror at what he had done.

I learned about this episode from Arnold himself. The day after the incident, he called me on the telephone and asked to come in to speak with me. He had done so on a few other occasions, so such a visit wasn't unusual, but he sounded especially anxious this time. When he arrived, we chatted for several minutes as I waited for him to bring up the topic for which he had come. Finally, he said he needed to talk about something I had mentioned to him in a previous conversation (I routinely discuss caregiver aggression in a general way with caregivers as part of my attempt to educate them about Alzheimer's disease, and also as a way to discreetly invite them to share their own experiences). He broke down and said he had slapped his wife, and that he was afraid he might do it again.

Immediately I assured him that although feeling guilty was normal, we would replace that feeling with action; namely, taking positive steps to alleviate the stress, frustration, and anger that had caused him to act out in the first place, and thus help prevent any future incidents. One step I had him take right away was to schedule more respite time for himself. He felt he needed to always be with Evelyn, so he was getting out of the house alone for only a few hours once a week. We arranged for his niece and a neighbor, both of whom Evelyn enjoyed, to come in once a week each for an entire afternoon so Arnold could visit friends, go to a museum, see a movie, or, one of his favorite activities that he had stopped doing because of Evelyn—spend time in the library.

We also discussed some diversionary tactics Arnold could take whenever Evelyn would repeat sentences or questions. If she kept asking the same question, say, "Where are we going?", instead of saying, "We're not going anywhere," he could respond by asking her a question: "Where do you want to go?" This approach—answering a question with a question—causes some people with Alzheimer's to break the cycle of asking questions and gets them to respond.

I believe it is essential that caregivers be allowed to talk without guilt about any acting out they do against their loved one. This is the first step toward getting them immediate help so such episodes don't happen again.

The real danger lies with those who don't reach out for assistance and who harbor their guilt along with the feelings that caused them to act out in the first place. Living with such emotions, along with the continued challenges caregiving brings, is a volatile situation that can result in unintentional harm to the patient. Organizations such as the Alzheimer's Association and various Alzheimer's support groups are good resources, as may be caring friends and family members (see the Appendix). The important thing is to seek help *immediately*, so that a solution—whether it be getting regular respite, finding part-time or full-time help, nursing home placement, or finding new ways to deal with the situation—can be found.

LETTING GO

I know that as a caregiver, you're concerned about the safety and well-being of your loved one. You also want him or her to be as independent and happy as possible, able to live life to the fullest. The problem is, often it seems as though these two goals are at odds. What if your loved one wants to do something you think is risky or foolish? What if that something is an activity that he or she used to engage in competently in the past, but now you're concerned? How do you know when to let go?

My general "rule" is, whatever keeps the patient motivated and happy, encourage it. Some slight modifications may be required to accommodate difficulties with memory or judgment. Flora had been a volunteer at her local library for more than twenty years. She spent ten to fifteen hours a week helping reshelve the books and set up displays. By the fifth year after her diagnosis, she was having difficulty following the numbers on the books to reshelve them, so the librarian asked her if she'd like to help with the children's story hour instead. Flora's daughter, Colleen, felt it was time for her mother to quit, but Flora desperately wanted to stay.

"She can't do what she used to," says Colleen. "I'm afraid she'll get confused someday and become upset. I just want to protect her." But rather than protect her mother, Colleen was smothering her. The library staff was willing and pleased to have Flora as a volunteer (they realized she was having memory problems, but were not informed of her diagnosis), and Flora felt useful and fulfilled.

Sometimes there are elements of danger to consider, but if you have taken responsible precautions, I see no reason to deprive a person who has Alzheimer's disease from pursuing their dreams. Jessica had a lifelong love of modern art, and she attended every gallery opening or new show she could. Her husband, Michael, typically accompanied her, but one night he announced that he didn't care to go. A half hour later, after Michael had fallen asleep in the recliner while reading, Jessica put on her coat and left the apartment. She hailed a cab, handed the driver a copy of the announcement about the gallery opening, and told him to take her there.

Michael didn't wake up until several hours later, and then discovered his wife was missing. Although he was worried, he also knew he had taken appropriate preventive measures. "She's registered with the Alzheimer's Association's Safe Return Program, so she wears an identifying bracelet and carries identification in her handbag," he says. "I also sewed her name, address, and phone number into all of her coats and sweaters." Michael immediately called the gallery and spoke with someone, who told him Jessica was there. He then pondered whether he should go get her or tell her to come home by herself. He chose the latter after securing a promise from his wife over the phone that she would leave immediately for home.

"I see it as a compromise," says Michael. "I don't want to restrict her to the house, and I don't want her to feel as if I'm baby-sitting her. As the disease progresses, I will likely be more restrictive with her, but I'll still want her to enjoy her art as much as possible and be as independent as possible. I'll just have to reach that balance."

SEXUAL RELATIONS

For many couples who enjoyed a sexual relationship before one of them developed Alzheimer's disease, continuing that relationship is important to them. If you are among that group, you may find that along with the desire often comes embarrassment and uncertainty about the "appropriateness" of your feelings. Is it "right" for you, the unaffected partner, to want to continue sexual relations with your loved one? Is there something "wrong" with you if you do? What if your partner wants sexual relations and you don't?

Sexuality is part of who we are as human beings, and I believe it is unrealistic and detrimental to a couple's relationship to sweep that part of their lives under the rug—unless they want to—because one partner has Alzheimer's disease. The question then becomes, where can the unaffected partner turn for help or advice about this issue?

Most people, including physicians, are not comfortable talking about the subject of sexual relations with their patients and patients' partners. Some people think it's even inappropriate for individuals who have Alzheimer's disease to be thinking about or engaging in sex at all. These conflicting feelings can make it difficult for caregivers to know what to do.

Olga, an attractive sixty-nine-year-old former teacher, had been feeling very guilty about still wanting to have sexual relations with her husband, Leonard, who had been diagnosed with Alzheimer's disease four years ago. She and Leonard had been married for nearly fifty years, and they had maintained a fairly active sex life until about two years ago, when Leonard, who is seventy-four, seemed to lose interest. Olga was hurt that her husband was turning away from her, yet at the same time she wondered if she was being selfish to want attention from him when he was feeling lost and confused.

"I didn't know who to talk to," she says. "I had been going to this support group for a few months, and I felt pretty comfortable with most of the people, especially a woman named Massie. One day Massie came up to me after our meeting and said she had to talk to somebody. Then she told me how terrible she felt that she still wanted sex with her husband, but he didn't. Then she cried, and I cried too, not just because I felt sorry for her but because I had found someone who knew what I had been going through! We talked for hours about it, and afterwards we both felt better.

"We both discovered too that we had been holding back from our husbands, really afraid to approach them physically and to let them know we needed physical contact. So Massie and I promised each other we would try to be more loving with our spouses and see if that helped. I must admit that now when I approach Leonard and hug him, he hugs me back, as he hasn't lost the need for a hug. Now we snuggle in bed and sometimes we have sex. I feel much better about our relationship. And Massie says she's noticed some improvement with her husband, too."

In my practice, I find that in most cases, spouses or partners don't directly bring up the subject of sexual relations, but they allude to it. That's my cue to introduce it into our conversation in a casual way, opening the door for discussion. If your doctor isn't receptive to talking about sexuality, or if you aren't comfortable discussing the topic with him or her, you might seek the services of a counselor who has experience dealing with the sexual concerns of handicapped individuals and/or people who have dementia. If you don't want to ask your doctor for a referral, you can contact your local Alzheimer's Association or a support group for one (see the Appendix).

WHOM DO YOU TELL?

This is a common question. Do you tell family and friends about your Alzheimer's disease? One patient of mine, a very independent man with early Alzheimer's, proposed telling his large group of friends about his diagnosis during his seventy-fourth birthday party celebration. The wife of a patient wanted to let their married friends know. I generally adopt the "don't ask, don't tell" policy. I find that most persons, even physicians, unconsciously adopt a more dismissive attitude toward the patient, talking in front of the person as though they were not there, not giving weight to their complaints, assuming that they always forget or that they are always wrong. This marginalization can actually make a person's condition worse.

I always believe that regardless of the stage of the illness, patients instinctively understand and dislike being patronized, even if it's done inadvertently. Families will often ask, "But how can I not tell anyone? It's obvious that there is a problem." People are rarely as observant as all that. It is only very late in the course of the condition that others become aware of a problem. I will then instruct families to say that the patient has a specific condition such as a language disorder or stroke, before using the term "Alzheimer's disease."

To illustrate how unobservant we can be sometimes, here is a personal example. With nearly a decade of experience in the field, I eat, think, and sleep memory disorders. One day I was out grocery shopping with my eight-year-old daughter when we struck up a conversation with a charming elderly gentleman in the produce aisle. He asked if we lived close by and I said yes. A couple of minutes later, after discussing the quality of the tomatoes, he casually asked whether we lived close by and I said yes again.

To make a long story short, in the course of a pleasant five-minute conversation, he had asked me the same question several times. When we moved on, I commented to my daughter about what a nice man he was and she looked at me, puzzled: "Mom," she said, "didn't you know he had a memory problem?" It all then clicked into place, the classic "cocktail personality" of some persons with early dementia in whose company you can spend hours without being aware of any problems. Here I was the memory "expert," completely taken in. So, "don't ask, don't tell." Believe me, it is better for all concerned. Despite this general rule, because patient and caregivers do feel isolated, I suggest taking one or two very select persons into your confidence and keeping them informed about what is happening. However, do let them know about your need for privacy in this matter.

THE BOTTOM LINE

The health and physical, emotional, and spiritual well-being of the caregivers of people who have Alzheimer's disease are of paramount importance, yet all too often they can be overlooked. My goal is always to keep both parties as fulfilled and healthy as possible, and that goal can be achieved when caregivers acknowledge that they have needs that must be met, and that meeting them is not selfish; and that they will have challenging emotional moments, and they too should be dealt with rather than suppressed. The most courageous thing caregivers can do is admit they need help, and then go after it.

Chapter 13

Looking Ahead: The Future of Alzheimer's Disease

Throughout this book, we have explored Alzheimer's disease from many angles—we have looked at the causes and risk factors, medical and alternative approaches to treatment of symptoms, creative ways to help preserve memory, and the concerns of caregivers. Our focus has been on the here and now, Alzheimer's disease as it is at this moment in time and how it impacts your life and that of your loved one today.

But there is another side to Alzheimer's disease. While you and millions of other caregivers and people with Alzheimer's disease live with the day-to-day realities of the disease—the joys and tears, the challenges and achievements—there are thousands of researchers and doctors working to find the cause and a cure for the disease. They are developing new drugs and new ways to deal with symptoms; they are working on hope.

Rarely a week goes by when there isn't at least one report of a new discovery concerning Alzheimer's disease, results of a new study, or some promising news about a new drug. For example, while I was writing this book, memantine, a promising drug I had been using in my practice for years as part of research studies, was approved by the Food and Drug Administration. In addition, scientists at Duke University Medical Center discovered a gene that may influence the age of onset of Alzheimer's disease. Knowing how this gene works could open new doors for ways to delay onset of the disease.

It seems as if the pace of the investigative work is picking up speed, and that's good news for the rapidly growing number of baby boomers, as well as those who have already been diagnosed with the disease. A wide range of possibilities are in various stages of development. Here are some of the most exciting and innovative approaches.

A MEMAPSIN 2 INHIBITOR

In people who have Alzheimer's disease, the beta-amyloid protein piles up and creates the plaques that are characteristic of the disease. Scientists have found that a brain enzyme called memapsin 2 is involved in the formation of plaques. Memapsin 2 works along with another enzyme (called gamma secretase) to release beta-amyloid from long protein chains. In healthy people, the body can eliminate these pieces of beta-amyloid and prevent them from accumulating. Therefore, some researchers have asked themselves, what if we change the way memapsin 2 acts in the brain? Could we then prevent plaque from forming?

To answer these questions, scientists at Oklahoma Medical Research Foundation have created an inhibitor that fools memapsin 2 into acting on what it "thinks" is the part of the protein chain that contains beta-amyloid. When the enzyme tries to release the beta-amyloid from the chain, the inhibitor stops the action. Once the enzyme is stopped, beta-amyloid can't be released, and plaques can't form.

Now scientists are trying to turn this inhibitor into a drug that could have the potential to manage—but not cure—Alzheimer's disease, much like antihypertension drugs manage high blood pressure or insulin manages diabetes. Even if research and studies go well, such a drug won't be available until at least 2010 because it is still in the beginning stages of development.

AN ALZHEIMER'S VACCINE

In 2000 and 2001, things looked promising for a new Alzheimer's disease vaccine. The vaccine, called AN-1792, consisted of the protein beta-amyloid, which, when injected into an animal or individual who has Alzheimer's disease, is supposed to prompt the body to make antibodies against the protein. This is how vaccines work.

Researchers had tested AN-1792 in mice, where it seemed to successfully remove beta-amyloid from the brains of mice that had Alzheimer's disease. Scientists then began trials in humans, and the initial reports were enthusiastic. Then, however, fifteen people developed inflammation in the brain, and the trials were stopped in January 2002.

An autopsy was performed on one of the affected patients involved in the trial, and the report was released in 2003. Experts found evidence that the vaccine had helped eliminate the protein beta-amyloid, but they also found evidence of meningoencephalitis, an inflammatory brain disease. Meningoencephalitis is not a characteristic of Alzheimer's disease, and so the scientists believe the vaccine was responsible for the condition. Several other autopsy samples have since become available from this study and reveal that the vaccine has consistently reduced the plaque deposits seen in Alzheimer's disease.

Given these encouraging findings, researchers hope to develop a safer and more effective vaccine in the near future.

HOMOCYSTEINE RESEARCH: THE VITAL TRIAL

Just how important is the role of homocysteine in Alzheimer's disease? Many experts think it's very important, and it's hoped that the results of the VITAL (VITamins to Slow Alzheimer's) Trial will answer the question definitively. Begun in January 2003, the VITAL Trial will follow the cognitive functioning of 400 individuals who have been diagnosed with Alzheimer's disease and who have been given either high doses of folic acid, vitamin B_6, and vitamin B_{12} (60 percent of the participants), or a placebo (40 percent of participants) over an eighteen-month period. As you'll recall these three vitamins have been shown to reduce homocysteine levels (see chapter 5).

Estimated completion for the trial is early 2006.

NERAMEXANE

The drug memantine was approved by the Food and Drug Administration in late 2003, and it may soon share the marketplace with another drug in the same category—neramexane. Like memantine (see chapter 7), neramexane helps regulate the activity of glutamate, a chemical involved in nerve cell communication and which is believed to have a role in damaging brain cells. In April 2003, the producers of neramexane began to recruit about 400 individuals who had been diagnosed with moderate to severe Alzheimer's disease for a 26-week study. Results of the trial are not expected until 2005.

Why do we need another drug like memantine? It's not unusual for people to respond better to one drug than to another in a given category, in terms of effectiveness and/or side effects. Thus the presence of more than one drug in a category offers patients treatment options.

CLIOQUINOL

In the 1970s, a drug called clioquinol (also known as clioquinoline) was removed from the market when it was linked to a rare neurological disorder. Recently, however, the drug has been studied to see how it helps eliminate beta-amyloid, the protein that creates the plaques associated with Alzheimer's disease. Studies in mice have been conducted by Ashley Bush of Harvard and his colleagues.

So far, researchers have found that the drug binds to two metals—copper and zinc—which are found in the plaque. These metals cause beta-amyloid to produce hydrogen peroxide, which destroys brain cells. When clioquinol attaches itself to the metals, it helps remove them from the brain, which then prevents brain cells from being destroyed. While this has been true in a significant number of mice that have been treated, whether this will hold true in humans is currently being investigated. Patients who are being given clioquinol are also receiving supplements of vitamin B_{12}, because one of the main side effects of clioquinol is that it depletes the body's reserves of this vitamin, causing neurotoxicity.

AMPAKINES

Since the early 1990s researchers have been studying a new class of drugs called ampakines. These drugs have the ability to enhance memory and cognition in a different way than do drugs in other categories that are used to treat Alzheimer's disease. Ampakines affect the activity of specific components (called AMPA receptors), which help compensate for a reduced output of glutamate in the brain. For now, ampakines are being tested in people who have mild cognitive impairment as well as those who have Alzheimer's disease.

COGNISHUNT

Some researchers believe that toxic substances, including fragments of beta-amyloid and tau proteins, may accumulate in the cerebrospinal fluid in people who have Alzheimer's disease and contribute to brain cell damage. To help remove those toxins, they are investigating the use of a shunt (trade name COGNIShunt), a device that can drain the cerebrospinal fluid and the toxic substances from the brain. This shunt is similar to one that is used to drain excess fluid from the brain in people who have hydrocephalus, a condition characterized by a buildup of cerebrospinal fluid in the brain that causes the head to enlarge.

To protect the brain, the empty spaces around and within it are filled with a protective substance called cerebrospinal fluid. Normally, the body continuously produces and absorbs this fluid, which helps maintain it at a healthy level. The effectiveness of this process declines with age, however, and for some people, excess toxins may accumulate rather than be drained away. This may be at least part of the reason Alzheimer's disease develops.

In October 2002, scientists reported on the results of a pilot study in which twenty-nine people with Alzheimer's disease participated. Fifteen of the patients received the shunt; fourteen did not. Over one year, symptoms of the disease stabilized in the patients who had the shunt and worsened in those who did not. Although these results seem encouraging, the study sample was too small to lead to any conclusions. Therefore, more trials and research are needed to determine whether this approach is safe and whether toxins in the cerebrospinal fluid contribute to the destruction of brain cells in Alzheimer's disease. One more consideration is the fact that implanting a shunt is a surgical procedure, and all surgery involves risks that must be weighed against potential benefits.

THE BOTTOM LINE

The few future potential treatments presented in this chapter represent only a fraction of those in the pipeline. Researchers around the world are conducting scores of experiments, trials, and studies of ways to diagnose, treat, and cure Alzheimer's disease. Many, if not most, of these efforts will never make it to market. But among those that do will hopefully be the one, or two, or more that make all the difference in the lives of the millions of people who have, and the millions of those who are predicted to get, Alzheimer's disease.

Glossary

acetylcholine: a neurotransmitter (chemical in the brain) that plays a major role in the transmission of signals between nerves that are responsible for memory and learning. People with Alzheimer's disease have very low levels of this chemical.

age-associated memory impairment: the type of memory changes that occur as part of the normal aging process without the presence of disease

ampakines: a class of drugs that increases the activity of certain chemicals in the brain that are involved in memory

amygdala: the area of the brain, located in the temporal lobe, that is involved in emotional memory and response

amyloid-beta: a type of protein that collects in the brain and forms deposits that contribute to the destruction of brain cells

amyloid plaque: a substance composed of beta-amyloid protein plus dead and dying brain cells. The plaque accumulates in the brain of people who have Alzheimer's disease.

antioxidant: a substance that helps stop the oxidative damage done by free radicals

ApoE4: a gene that has been implicated in increasing the risk of developing Alzheimer's disease

apraxia: an inability to perform learned movements or activities for reasons other than impaired motor strength, comprehension, or coordination

cerebral cortex: the part of the brain that is involved in language, reasoning, learning, and other high-functioning processes

cholinesterase inhibitors: medications that help preserve levels of the neurotransmitter acetylcholine and thus help maintain cognitive functioning

clioquinol (or clioquinoline): an antibiotic that may prove useful in removing plaques from the brain. It is under investigation.

cognitive function: higher-level mental activities such as remembering, reasoning, abstract thought, speaking, reading, writing, and making decisions

cortisol: a steroid hormone secreted by the adrenal glands in response to psychological or physical stress

delusion: a false idea that usually arises from misinterpretation of a situation or an event, but one which the individual firmly believes is true even though there is no evidence to support the belief

dementia: a general term used to describe any irreversible condition characterized by a decline in mental abilities due to nerve cell death; for example, the damage to brain cells caused by amyloid plaque deposits seen in Alzheimer's disease

donepezil (Aricept): a cholinesterase inhibitor drug used to treat Alzheimer's disease

dopamine: a neurotransmitter in the brain that, when present in normal quantities, helps many critical brain functions. When out of balance, it can cause brain dysfunction and disease.

estrogen: a naturally occurring hormone that appears to play a major role in Alzheimer's disease and that may reduce the risk of developing the disease when given to postmenopausal women

folic acid: a nutrient (one of the B vitamins) that appears to be helpful in preventing Alzheimer's disease. Also known as folate.

free radicals: molecules that can cause oxidative stress, which leads to cell damage, accelerated aging, and chronic diseases such as Alzheimer's, cancer, and diabetes

frontal lobe: the front part of the brain. It is involved in controlling abilities such as coordinating thoughts, planning, and scheduling.

galantamine (Reminyl): a cholinesterase inhibitor drug used to treat Alzheimer's disease

ginkgo biloba: a Chinese herb that may be helpful in treating memory loss

glutamate: a chemical (neurotransmitter) involved in learning and memory

hippocampus: an area deep in the temporal lobe of the brain that is involved in memory and learning

hydergine: a substance derived from a fungus that has yielded mixed results when used to treat memory loss. It has properties similar to those of cholinesterase inhibitors.

immediate memory: memory for sounds, sights, smells, and other sensory stimuli that lasts for less than a second before it goes into short-term memory

lecithin: a substance found in all cells that some people take as a supplement to help improve memory, but which has not demonstrated good results

long-term memory: memory that has become relatively permanent

melatonin: a hormone, secreted by the pineal gland, that regulates immune function, mood, the sleep-wake cycle, and sexual behavior

memantine (Namenda): a drug that affects certain brain receptors (N-methyl-D-aspartate) and has proven helpful in treating Alzheimer's disease

mild cognitive impairment: a condition that causes slight problems with memory and other cognitive functions, but not serious enough to impair a person's ability to live independently

Mini-Mental State Exam: a standard, 30-point mental examination often given to measure an individual's basic cognitive skills, such as writing, language, orientation, and memory

mitochondria: organs within cells that are responsible for producing energy

mnemonists: memory specialists who use emotion to help them remember

neuron: a brain or nerve cell

neurotransmitter: a chemical substance that helps neurons communicate with one another

oxidative stress: the damage inflicted upon the cells by free radicals as oxygen interacts with other substances in the body

parietal lobe: the area of the brain located above and behind the temporal lobe

Parkinson's disease: a progressive neurological disease in which nerve cells in specific parts of the brain die for reasons unknown. Symptoms typically include tremors, difficulties with movement, speech impediments, and dementia in the later stages of the disease.

phosphatidylserine: a nutrient taken as a supplement to help treat memory impairment

rivastigmine (Exelon): a cholinesterase inhibitor drug used to treat Alzheimer's disease

selegiline (Eldepryl): a drug with antioxidant effects that helps delay functional decline in people who have Alzheimer's disease

serotonin: a neurotransmitter found in abnormally low levels in people who have Alzheimer's disease and in individuals who have depression

short-term memory: memory that lasts for only a few minutes

statins: drugs typically used to reduce high cholesterol levels. They may also be useful in reducing the risk of Alzheimer's disease.

tacrine (Cognex): a cholinesterase inhibitor used to treat Alzheimer's disease. Because it can cause serious side effects and must be taken frequently, tacrine is rarely used today.

tangles: also known as neurofibrillary tangles; an accumulation of abnormal hair-like protein clumps in nerve cells

tau protein: the main protein that makes up the tangles found in people who have Alzheimer's disease

vitamin E: an antioxidant that, when taken in high doses, may help delay loss of cognitive functioning associated with aging

References and Suggested Readings

Ahlgrimm, Maria, RPh, et al. *The HRT Solution: A Comprehensive, Personalized Program of Natural Hormone Replacement to Relieve Menopausal Symptoms and Restore Vitality, Sexuality, and Health for Life.* 2nd ed. New York: Avery Penguin Putnam, 2003.

The Caregiver Newsletter. Available through Duke University Medical Center, Duke Family Support Program; 919-660-7510.

Cordrey, C. *Hidden Treasures: Music and Memory Activities for People with Alzheimer's.* Mt. Airy, MD: ElderSong Publications, 1994.

Davidson, A. *Alzheimer's: A Love Story: One Year in My Husband's Journey.* Secaucus, NJ: Carol Publishing, 1997.

Devi, Gayatri. *Estrogen, Memory, and Menopause: 136 Questions and Answers on the Symptoms and Treatment of Hormone Related Memory and Mood Disorders.* New York: AlphaSigma Books, 2000.

Devi, Gayatri. *Exercises for a Healthy Brain* (CD-ROM). Available through www.nymemory.org.

Dowling, J. R. *Keeping Busy: A Handbook of Activities for*

Persons with Dementia. Baltimore, MD: Johns Hopkins University Press, 1995.

Goldstein, Steven R., and Laurie Ashner. *The Estrogen Alternative.* New York: Putnam, 1998.

Hodgson, Harriet. *Alzheimer's—Finding the Words: A Communication Guide for Those Who Care.* New York: John Wiley, 1995.

Knowles, Carrie. *The Last Childhood: A Family Story of Alzheimer's.* New York: Three Rivers Press, 2000.

Kuhn, Daniel, MSW. *Alzheimer's Early Stages: First Steps in Caring and Treatment.* Alameda, CA: Hunter House, 1999.

Loverde, Joy. *The Complete Eldercare Planner: Where to Start, Which Questions to Ask, and How to Find Help.* New York: Times Books, 2000.

Mace, N. L., and P. V. Rabins. *The 36-Hour Day: A Family Guide to Caring for Persons with Alzheimer's Disease, Related Dementing Illnesses, and Memory Loss in Later Life.* 3rd ed. Baltimore, MD: Johns Hopkins University Press, 1999.

Medina, John J., PhD. *What You Need to Know about Alzheimer's Disease.* Oakland, CA: New Harbinger, 1999.

Northrup, Christiane. *The Wisdom of Menopause.* New York: Bantam, 2003.

Schwartz, Erika, MD. *The 30-Day Natural Hormone Plan: Look and Feel Young Again—Without Synthetic HRT.* New York: Warner Books, 2004.

Shanks, Lela Knox. *Your Name Is Hughes Hannibal Shanks: A Caregiver's Guide to Alzheimer's.* New York: Penguin, 1999.

Shenk, David. *The Forgetting: Alzheimer's: Portrait of an Epidemic.* New York: Doubleday, 2001.

Small, Gary, MD. *The Memory Bible.* New York: Hyperion, 2002.

Snowdon, David, PhD. *Aging with Grace: What the Nun Study Teaches Us about Leading Longer, Healthier, and More Meaningful Lives.* New York: Bantam, 2001.

Snyder, L. *Speaking Our Minds: Personal Reflections from Individuals with Alzheimer's Disease.* New York: W. H. Freeman, 1999.

Tanzi, Rudolph E., and Ann B. Parson. *Decoding Darkness: The Search for the Genetic Causes of Alzheimer's Disease.* New York: Perseus, 2001.

Today's Caregiver Magazine. Available through www.caregiver.com; also 800-829-2734.

Wells, Suzanne, ed., and the American Horticultural Therapy Association. *Horticultural Therapy and the Older Adult Population.* Binghamton, NY: Haworth Press, 1977.

Appendix

ASSOCIATIONS AND OTHER RESOURCES

Alliance for Children and Families
11700 West Lake Park Drive
Milwaukee, WI 53224-3099
414-359-1040
www.alliance1.org

Alzheimer's Association (national headquarters)
225 N. Michigan Avenue, Floor 17
Chicago, IL 60611-1676
800-272-3900
www.alz.org

Alzheimer's Disease Education and Referral Center (ADEAR)
PO Box 8250
Silver Spring, MD 20907-8250
800-438-4380
www.alzheimers.org

Alzheimer's Prevention Foundation International
2420 N. Pantano Road

Tucson, AZ 85715
520-749-8374
www.Alzheimersprevention.org

American Association for Geriatric Psychiatry
7910 Woodmont Avenue, Suite 1050
Bethesda, MD 20814-3004
301-654-7850
www.aagpgpa.org

American Board of Medical Specialties
1007 Church Street, Suite 404
Evanston, IL 60201-5913
Phone verification: 866-ASK-ABMS
www.abms.org

Family Caregiver Alliance
690 Market Street, Suite 600
San Francisco, CA 94104
415-434-3388
www.caregiver.org

National Academy of Elder Law Attorneys, Inc.
1604 North Country Club Road
Tucson, AZ 85716
520-881-4005
www.naela.org

National Council on the Aging
300 D Street SW, Suite 801
Washington, DC 20024
202-479-1200
www.ncoa.org

National Council on Women's Health, Inc.
445 East 69th Street, Suite 320
New York, NY 10021
212-746-6967

National Institute of Mental Health (NIMH)
Office of Communications
6001 Executive Boulevard, Room 8184, MSC 9663
Bethesda, MD 20892-9663
301-443-4513
www.nimh.nih.gov

National Institute on Aging
Building 31, Room 5C27
31 Center Drive, MSC 2292
Bethesda, MD 20892
301-496-1752
www.nia.nih.gov

SUPPORT GROUPS/CHAT ROOMS/E-MAIL SUPPORT

Alzheimer's Association
800-272-3900
www.alz.org

Alzheimer's Disease Education and Referral Center (ADEAR)
800-438-4380
www.alzheimers.org

Alzheimer's Support (chat room)
www.alzheimersupport.com/Chat
www.alzwell.com
Caregiver support Web site with a newsletter, Q&A, articles, resource lists, message board

Caregivers' Forum from Third Age (support and chat)
http://thirdage.com/family

Children of Aging Parents
800-227-7294
www.caps4caregivers.org

Dr. C. Everett Koop's Chat
www.drkoop.com/_mem_bin/FormsLogin.asp?

ElderCare Neighborhood Network (support and chat room)
www.ec-online.net/Community/Neighborhood/Neighborhood.html
www.ec-online.net/chat.htm

Friends and Relatives of Institutionalized Aged
212-732-4455
www.fria.org

A Little Heart to Heart (chat room)
www.zarcrom.com/users/alzheimers

National Association of Home Care
202-547-7424
www.nahc.org

Well Spouse Foundation
800-838-0879
www.wellspouse.org

MEMORY DISORDER CLINICS

For a list of more than one hundred memory disorder clinics across the United States, see www.caregiving-solutions.com/rescen.html. This Web site lists memory disorder clinics by state and gives contact information as well as links to Web sites for each clinic when available. Most states are represented. If you do not see a memory disorder clinic near you, ask your physician for a recommendation or contact your local Alzheimer's Association office. You may also contact Alzheimer Solutions (the organization that provides the list of U.S. memory disorder clinics on the caregiving-solutions Web site) at 3122 Knorr Street, Philadelphia, PA 19149; 215-624-2098.

PRODUCTS

These suppliers, as well as others not listed, offer products that can help ensure the safety and comfort of people who have Alzheimer's disease. Some of the products they offer include doorknob covers, temperature sensors, door barriers, room monitors, glow tape, grab bars, electrical outlet covers, ID bracelets, and items to make mealtimes easier (e.g., suction cup plates, double-handled cups, drinking aids, sectioned plates). Hardware stores, large children's specialty stores, and medical supply facilities may carry some of these items as well.

www.agelessdesign.com
http://edenalt.safeshopper.com
www.caregiving-solutions.com/safetyitems.html
www.organicbebe.com/safety_locks.asp

Index

Page numbers of illustrations appear in italics.

About the Author

Gayatri Devi, M.D., believes passionately that a dignified, fulfilling life is possible for Alzheimer's patients and their families.

Dr. Devi is director of the New York Memory Services, where 60 percent of the patients under her care have Alzheimer's disease. She is also a former director of the Memory Disorders Center at the Center for Women's Health at Columbia Presbyterian Eastside and former co-director of the Clinical Core of Columbia University's Alzheimer's Disease Research Center. She has also served as spokesperson for the New York chapter of the Alzheimer's Association.

With board certifications in both neurology and psychiatry, Dr. Devi is well equipped to handle both the psychological and neurological aspects of this complex disease.

Dr. Devi's extensive experience with all stages of the disease, her unrelenting belief that a comprehensive blend of conventional and complementary methods can significantly improve the lives of Alzheimer's patients, and her optimistic outlook make this book truly unique.

Dr. Devi is also the author of *Estrogen, Memory, and Menopause.*

FIBROMYALGIA FATIGUE

The Powerful Program That Helps You Boost Your Energy and Reclaim Your Life

GLAUCOMA

The Essential Treatments and Advances That Could Save Your Sight

HIP AND KNEE REPLACEMENT SURGERY

Everything You Need to Know to Make the Right Decisions

HPV AND ABNORMAL PAP SMEARS

Get the Facts on This Dangerous Virus—Protect Your Health and Your Life!

HYPERTENSION

The Revolutionary Nutrition and Lifestyle Program to Help Fight High Blood Pressure

HYPOTHYROIDISM

A Simple Plan for Extraordinary Results

IBS

Eliminate Your Symptoms and Live a Pain-free, Drug-free Life

KNEE PAIN AND SURGERY

Learn the Truth About MRIs and Common Misdiagnoses—and Avoid Unnecessary Surgery

MENOPAUSE
The Breakthrough Book on *Natural* Hormone Balance

MIGRAINES
The Breakthrough Program That Can Help End Your Pain

OSTEOPOROSIS
Help Prevent—and Even Reverse—the Disease That Burdens Millions of Women

PARKINSON'S DISEASE
A Holistic Program for Optimal Wellness

PEDIATRIC FIBROMYALGIA
A Safe, New Treatment Plan for Children

PREMENOPAUSE
Balance Your Hormones and Your Life from Thirty to Fifty

SINUSITUS
Relieve Your Symptoms and Identify the Real Source of Your Pain